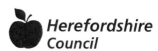

# A DAD'S GUIDE
# TO HAVING A BABY

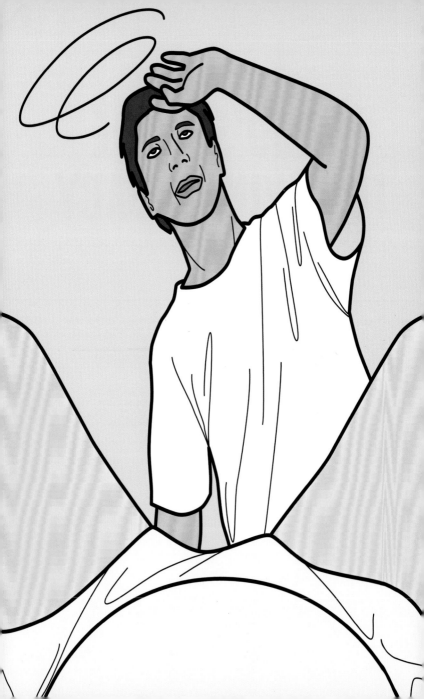

# A DAD'S GUIDE TO HAVING A BABY

Everything a new dad needs
to know about pregnancy
and caring for a newborn

## DOMINIC BLISS

DOG 'n' BONE

**Thanks to my lovely daughters Daisy and Lola (it's been a steep learning curve!), and my wonderful wife Sally.**

This third edition published in 2019 by Dog 'n' Bone Books
An imprint of Ryland Peters & Small Ltd
20–21 Jockey's Fields          341 E 116th St
London WC1R 4BW              New York, NY 10029

www.rylandpeters.com

10 9 8 7 6 5 4 3 2 1

First edition published as *A Man's Guide to Having a Baby* in 2013 by Dog 'n' Bone Books

Text © Dominic Bliss 2019
Design and illustration © Dog 'n' Bone Books 2019

A CIP catalog record for this book is available from the Library of Congress and the British Library.

ISBN: 978 1 911026 82 2

Printed in China

Editor: Marion Paull
Design concept: Geoff Borin
Spread design: Emma Forge
and Jerry Goldie (pages 110–125)
Cover design: Emily Breen
Illustration: Kuo Kang Chen

Please note that the advice in this book is not to be considered as a substitute for medical advice from your family doctor or any other qualified medical practitioner. If you treat yourself with natural medicines, such as herbs, you should always inform your doctor, because these can be very powerful and can interact with prescribed and over-the-counter medications.

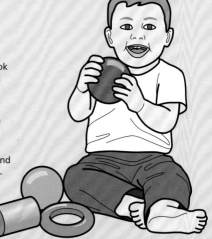

# Contents

# INTRODUCTION

# **CONGRATULATIONS**

So, your partner's pregnant. You've probably already completed your headless-chicken panicky run around the living room and, right now, you need some no-nonsense advice on how to be a thoroughly responsible dad.

Well, you've come to the right place. This book will give you all the practical advice you need to survive pregnancy (remember, you're pregnant, too), childbirth, and the first year of your baby's life.

Nowadays, modern dads are more involved in pregnancy and birth than ever before in human history. It's a role you should relish. Some of it will be straightforward and involve common sense; some of it will be fun; and some of it will be downright scary. But at no time will it be boring. Pregnancy and fatherhood are all part of life's rich pageant.

In this book, I concentrate on the factors that will most affect you, as a father. These include the essentials you need to know about what's happening to your partner's body and the baby inside her, but we will skim over the exclusively female aspects of pregnancy. Besides, there are countless books aimed at mothers that cover that kind of stuff—so, not so much about food cravings and sore nipples, but lots on catching the baby, changing diapers, and buying a stroller.

Throughout the book I use the term "partner" to refer to the woman who's carrying your baby. It's not the ideal term, I know. She may be your "wife," your "girlfriend," or even a one-night stand that got a little too amorous. "Partner" is simply a catch-all description.

Also, a quick note on the use of pronouns may be helpful. When I say "he," I'm referring to your baby; when I say "she," I mean your partner. This avoids confusion and makes sense since no women should be reading this book. Of course, there's a good chance you don't yet know the sex of your future offspring. If "he" turns out to be a "she," I apologize in advance.

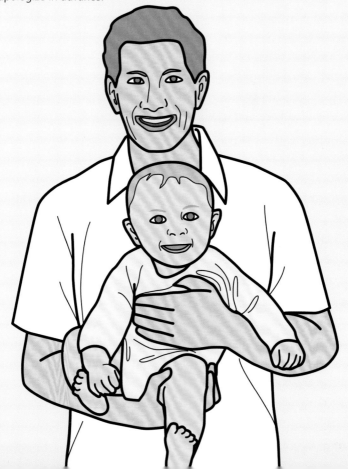

# No more baby jargon!

Trimesters and Braxton Hicks? Come again? When a bunch of parents-to-be gets together to talk about babies, some of us dads get decidedly uneasy. It can sound like they're all speaking a foreign language. Things get even more confusing once medical staff and hospitals wade in. Take control of all that jargon and find out what the hell they're jabbering on about. Welcome to the idiot's guide to technical terms used in pregnancy and baby care.

## A to Z of baby jargon

### A

**Amniocentesis:** The extraction of amniotic fluid to test for genetic abnormalities.

**Amniotic fluid:** The fluid that surrounds the baby and protects him while he's in the womb.

### B

**Babinski reflex:** Stroking the baby's foot causes the big toe to rise and the other toes to fan out.

**Baby blues:** A mild depression that many women feel in the days after giving birth.

**Blastocyst:** The ball of cells that later develops into the embryo.

**Braxton Hicks contractions:** Contractions that occur a little while before childbirth as the uterus gets ready for the real thing.

### C

**Cervix:** The lower, narrow end of the uterus where it joins with the top of the vagina.

**CNM:** A certified nurse-midwife.

**Contraction:** A tightening of the uterus, which thins and dilates the mother's cervix.

**Couvade syndrome:** A condition in which the father feels physical symptoms of pregnancy.

**Cradle cap:** A crusty skin rash that appears on the baby's scalp.

**C-section or cesarean:** The surgical procedure used to deliver a baby through the mother's abdomen.

# D

**Doula:** A maternity nurse, not necessarily trained.

**Down's syndrome:** A chromosomal condition resulting in birth defects.

# E

**Ectopic pregnancy:** The embryo implants outside the uterus.

**Endometrium:** The lining of the uterus.

**Epidural:** Pain relief injected into the mother's lower back during childbirth.

# F

**Forceps delivery:** The gentle use of two tongs to pull the baby's head out of the mother's vagina while she pushes.

# G

**Gestational diabetes:** A form of diabetes that some women develop during pregnancy.

**Gestational hypertension:** When a woman develops high blood pressure after 20 weeks of pregnancy.

# H

**Hypnobirthing:** Hypnotherapy to ease childbirth.

# I

**IVF:** In vitro fertilization, when the egg is fertilized by sperm outside of the woman's body.

# M

**Mastitis:** An infection of the mother's breast.

**Meconium:** The greenish-black first poo that a baby produces after birth.

**Meningitis:** Inflammation of the membranes covering the brain and spinal cord.

**Midwife:** The healthcare professional who supports the mother during birth.

**Miscarriage:** When a woman loses the baby during the first 20 weeks of pregnancy.

**Mongolian spot:** Black or blue marks on a newborn baby's legs or bottom.

# O

**OB/GYN:** Obstetrician/gynecologist, medical professionals trained in women's reproduction.

**Oligohydramnios:** A condition in which there is too little amniotic fluid in the uterus.

**Ovulation:** The phase in a woman's menstrual cycle when a mature egg is available to be fertilized.

# P

**Pertussis:** See Whooping cough, page 68.

**Pica:** A disorder that causes pregnant women to eat unusual substances, such as coal or starch.

**Placenta:** The organ that connects the fetus to the wall of the uterus and provides life support.

**Placenta previa:** The placenta implants too low on the wall of the uterus, near the cervix.

**Plagiocephaly:** Flattened head syndrome in the baby caused by his position in the womb or, once he's born, by resting his head on the same spot while asleep.

**Polyhydramnios:** A condition in which there is too much amniotic fluid in the uterus.

**Postpartum (or postnatal) depression:** A clinical depression that affects some mothers after childbirth.

**Postpartum (or postnatal) psychosis:** A more serious, and potentially lethal, version of postpartum depression.

**Pre-eclampsia:** When the mother has high blood pressure and protein in her urine.

**Pregnancy-induced hypertension (PIH):** See Gestational hypertension.

**Preterm birth:** A premature birth less than 37 weeks into the pregnancy.

# S

**SIDS:** Sudden infant death syndrome, also known as crib (or cot) death.

**Spina bifida:** A congenital disorder in which the spinal vertebrae do not fully form.

# T

**Trimester:** One of the three 12-week stages of pregnancy.

# U

**Ultrasound:** A sound pressure wave used to create a picture of the fetus growing in the womb.

**Uterus:** The mother's womb where the fetus grows.

# V

**Vacuum extraction:** A rounded cup is applied to the baby's head and vacuum pressure used to pull him out of the vagina while the mother pushes.

**Ventouse:** See Vacuum extraction.

**Vernix:** The white, waxy substance that coats a baby's skin when he is first born.

# W

**Weaning:** Transitioning a baby from milk to solid food.

# Z

**Zygote:** The earliest stage of an embryo.

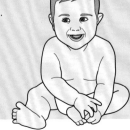

# The daddy suitability quiz

Find out whether you'll make a great first-time father. Take our multiple-choice daddy test.

### What's the best cure for morning sickness?

**a)** Hair of the dog

**b)** A lump of coal

**c)** Ginger infusion and a plain piece of toast

### Where might you perform a perineal massage?

**a)** Balls of her feet

**b)** Back of her neck

**c)** Between her vagina and bottom

### Braxton Hicks is the name for:

**a)** Your cousins living in Oklahoma

**b)** An alternative rock band from Ireland

**c)** Phantom contractions

### What does she mean by "My waters have broken"?

**a)** Her hot-water bottle is faulty.

**b)** The bath has overflowed.

**c)** The baby's amniotic sac has broken and leaked fluid out of her vagina.

### How do you get to hospital quickly?

**a)** I have a tandem bicycle. Mom can go on the back.

**b)** It's only a few stops by bus.

**c)** I've had a helipad installed on our roof.

**It's called a cesarean because:**

**a)** Afterward, her midriff looks a bit like a Caesar chicken salad.

**b)** Julius Caesar was the first person to be born in this way.

**c)** It's from the Latin verb "caedere," to cut.

**Your idea of a great weekend is:**

**a)** Sex, drugs, and rock 'n' roll

**b)** Video games and take-out pizza

**c)** Playgrounds and ballpits

**You've chosen a name for your baby based on what?**

**a)** The inspiration was Star Wars.

**b)** The name of the town where he was conceived.

**c)** You prefer to stick with the classics.

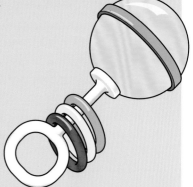

**What's on TV, Junior?**

**a)** The Texas Chainsaw Massacre

**b)** Playboy TV

**c)** Disney Channel

**What's for lunch?**

**a)** Raw oysters

**b)** Caviar and Champagne

**c)** Mashed banana and apple purée

## Your score:

**Mainly As:** Get yourself to antenatal classes!

**Mainly Bs:** Don't be surprised if your partner checks up on everything you do.

**Mainly Cs:** Hey, Superdad! Baby's safe in your hands.

# PART 1
# THE PREGNANCY

## There's a bun in the oven!

Perhaps you were both planning the pregnancy. Maybe you've been trying for a baby for months. Or maybe it was a complete shock for both of you and you're still reeling from the news.

Whichever way you learn of your new role as a father, it's important you reassure your partner with some sort of positive reaction. Sure, as she steps out of the bathroom brandishing her blue testing stick, she'll expect some initial emotions from you—tears, fainting, swearing, even startled-rabbit alarm. But once you're thinking straight again, you need to act the keen, responsible father (even if you're tempted to book that next flight to South America.)

**Why not celebrate straightaway?** Go out and buy a bottle of Champagne and some flowers and tell her how happy you are to be embarking on the next great stage of life together. The Champagne's for you; the flowers are for her.

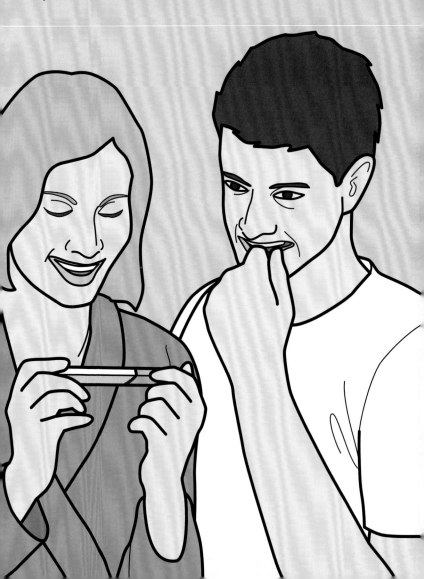

# Overcoming fear of fatherhood

Yes, it's a daunting prospect, up there with running the country, undergoing a heart transplant, and flying to Mars. But unlike politics, surgery, and space travel, it's a totally normal part of life. We men have been doing it since we were swinging through the trees.

Granted, an unplanned pregnancy is a lot harder to get your head around than a planned one. But there are advantages as well as disadvantages to parenthood.

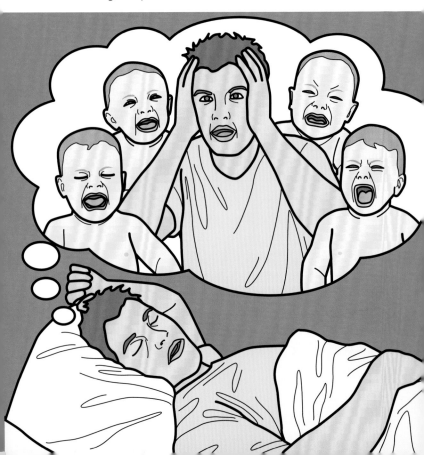

- I'll have less free time! Yes, but the free time I enjoy with my kids will—with a bit of planning—be just as enriching.

- My single friends will abandon me! Maybe. But I'll make new friends with the other dads at nursery and infant school.

- A child will be a drain on our financial resources! But I won't be going out as much so I'll save money that way.

- My career will suffer! But I'll use the life skills I learn as a father to further myself as an employee.

- Sleep deprivation will kill me! But I'm determined to help my baby into a good sleep routine. And I can sleep when he sleeps.

- Our sex life is over! But only for a short period. Then we'll both work hard to reinvigorate things in the bedroom.

- I'm just not cut out to be a father! No one really is. Men adapt to fill their new shoes.

- My wife has disappeared and been replaced by a mother! But I will make sure we have lots of non-baby time together.

## When to announce the pregnancy

If you're excited about the baby, the temptation is to blurt the news to your friends and family straightaway. And if you're daunted, you may need to discuss the prospects with someone close. Hold your horses, though. Around a fifth of all pregnancies end in miscarriage—often during the first 12 weeks. Announce it early and you risk going through the nightmare of having to tell everyone the tragic news. Much better (and more usual) to wait until you've had the first ultrasound scan (normally at 12 weeks) and you know the baby is healthy. Then you can text everyone and announce it on Facebook.

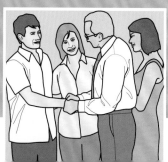

# Ultrasound scans

Healthy mothers tend to have two ultrasound scans, one at around
12 weeks to determine the due date and to screen for abnormalities,
and one at around 20 weeks to check that the fetus is developing
well. But some hospitals will operate different schedules. To help get
a good picture, it's a good idea for the mother to drink plenty of water
before the scan.

For both scans, the operator will start off by rubbing gel on
your partner's tummy to help the transmission of sound waves. Then

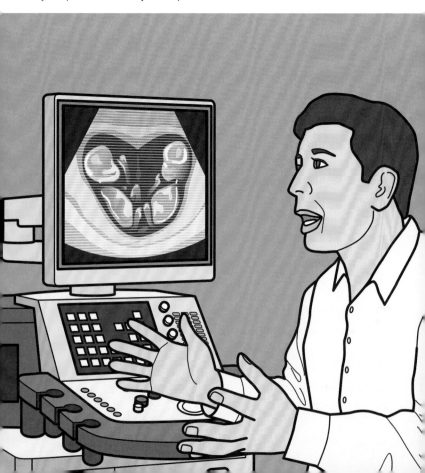

he'll move the transducer over the bump, which produces an image (a sonogram) on the screen.

Don't expect a pin-sharp image of your future child. At the first scan, the baby will look a bit like a small vegetable. At the second, depending on the angle at which he's lying in the womb, he can resemble anything from a monkey to an alien. You should get a chance to hear the heartbeat and see the limbs moving around.

Ask the ultrasound operator for a print-out of the image (there may be a charge). This is the first of millions of photos of your child. You can give it pride of place on the first page of your family photograph album.

## Scans check crucial information about your baby:

● Measuring the baby will confirm your partner's due date.

● Is the baby developing normally?

● Are you having twins? (Aaaghh!)

● Are there risks of abnormalities such as Down's syndrome or spina bifida?

● Is the baby lying in a good position for delivery?

## Should you reveal the gender?

At the second scan, the ultrasound operator will ask whether you want to know if it's a boy or a girl. (The first scan is too early to identify.) Many parents can't resist. If you're keen to get started on painting the baby's bedroom or choosing names, then prior knowledge is useful, although a surprise can be fun. No gender test is 100 percent accurate.

There is actually a psychological advantage to not finding out. With a possible 48 hours of labor on the cards, the eventual discovery of your baby's gender can be a goal for your exhausted partner to aim for, and a wonderful, life-affirming moment for both of you.

Ultrasound operators prefer to use "he" or "she" rather than the soulless "it." Don't take this as an unintentional indication of gender. Do get worried, however, if the operator uses "they."

And what if you want to know the gender but your partner doesn't? Here's a compromise. Ask the operator to write the answer on a piece of paper and place it in an envelope. Should temptation prove too great, one or both of you can break the seal at a later date.

## Jesus! We're having twins! Triplets!

The chances of giving birth to twins or triplets used to be fairly small, but thanks to modern fertilization techniques, such as IVF—now so popular across the western world— the odds have risen enormously.

There are two types of twins: identical (one zygote splits and forms two embryos) and fraternal (two separate eggs are fertilized by two separate sperms). Since there's less room in the mother's womb for each fetus, multiple births normally occur earlier than singleton births—three weeks earlier for twins, and six weeks earlier for triplets.

While there's a certain economy of scale to having multiples, don't doubt that you'll have your hands full. The good news is there's lots of help available. Why not join a local support group?

# Your partner's changing body

It's a bump, and it gets bigger every day … Right? Unfortunately, things are a lot more complicated than that. Pregnancy will have major ramifications on your partner's entire body and, of course, on her hormones. As the dad, it's a good idea to know what's going on. The more you learn about her body, the more you, personally, will feel confident about the pregancy.

Pregnancy is traditionally split into three trimesters—periods of approximately three months lasting from conception to birth.

The first trimester (from conception to week 12) is the least obvious. Your partner's body won't change massively but her breasts will. The good news is they'll get bigger. The bad news is that they will be very tender (sometimes painful) when touched. The areolas around the nipples will get darker and develop nodules. Your partner may well suffer from morning sickness (see page 29) and/or food cravings (see page 30), and will certainly be extremely tired because much of her energy is diverted to growing the fetus. As her uterus grows bigger, it presses against her bladder, making her have to pee much more often. Be ready to make extra stops on car journeys; have your finger poised over the pause button when watching DVDs; expect to be woken several times during the night.

It's only by the second trimester that you will notice your partner gaining weight and actually appearing pregnant to the outside world. Physical side effects include heartburn, constipation, thicker and shinier hair, a glowing complexion, and (wait for it!) an increase in libido.

The third trimester (the last 12 weeks) are the business end of the pregnancy. Your partner's bump will be reaching full size, restricting her movement and sleep. As the growing fetus puts pressure on her diaphragm, she will find herself short of breath. High blood pressure can lead to puffy hands, wrists, ankles, and feet. In later stages, she may even get Braxton Hicks contractions (see page 8).

# Your baby's changing body

Wouldn't it be great if the bump was see-through? A womb with a view, so to speak. Then you could observe your baby's physical development perfectly.

Unfortunately, a bit of imagination is required. In the later stages, you'll feel him kicking (and even his heartbeat), but until then it's a waiting game.

### First 6 weeks
(The size of a lentil)
After conception, the fertilized egg grows into a ball of cells (blastocyst), which implants itself in the lining of the uterus. By week six, the embryo looks like a cross between a shrimp and a baked bean. The heart and spinal cord begin to develop, and rudimentary limbs start to sprout.

### Weeks 7 to 10
(The size of a baked bean)
It's now that the embryo finally starts to resemble a tiny human (or E.T., perhaps.) All the internal organs are there, fingers and toes are visible, the face and its features start to develop, limbs grow, as do teeth buds. His head looks too big for his body as the brain enlarges. The tail he had as a tiny embryo disappears. His skin is covered with downy hair.

### Weeks 11 to 14
(The size of a golf ball)
His bones start developing. Fingernails and toenails have formed. Genital organs grow. He starts drinking amniotic fluid and excreting it as urine. He can now move his body and do hiccups.

The entries below can be used as a guideline to how your baby is developing in the womb. So when you are at the local bar at week 8, panicking about how the new baby will change your life, you can find comfort in the fact that the peanut you are munching on is rougly the size of the baby in your partner's body.

## Weeks 15 to 18
(The size of an iPhone)
Ears and tastebuds start to function. The lungs are developing.

## Weeks 19 to 26
(The size of an American football)
His skin becomes sensitive to touch so that he moves if there is pressure on the abdomen. He now has sleeping and waking cycles.

## Weeks 27 to 30
(The size of an iPad)
He wriggles and kicks.

## Weeks 31 to 34
(The size of a small backpack)
His eyes can now focus and blink. There's lots of hair on his head.

## Weeks 35 to 40
(The size of a … well, a baby)
He is fully mature, very snug inside the womb. His body is plump. Inside his intestine is a dark substance called meconium, which he will excrete after birth.

# Mother medical issues

While most pregnancies run pretty smoothly, the mother may face various discomforts or even complications. In those circumstances, you need to be aware of what's happening.

## Common complaints during pregnancy

Here are some common issues to look out for.

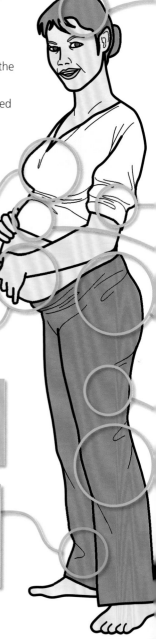

**Sore breasts:** They may be getting bigger but they can be sore all through the pregnancy.

**Morning sickness:** See page 29.

**Braxton Hicks:** These contractions normally occur late in the pregnancy as the mother's body gets ready for the real thing.

**Water retention:** Many pregnant women get swollen ankles, feet, and hands. Suddenly that expensive engagement ring you gave her is too small for her to wear.

**Mood swings:** Hormonal changes can turn your lovely girl into a crazed banshee, especially as the birth approaches. Bear with her.

**Insomnia:** The baby doesn't always sleep when the mother wants to.

**Fainting:** With so much blood going to the womb, often too little reaches the mother's head. She should avoid standing up too quickly.

**Backache:** It's not surprising this is a problem, given the extra human being living inside her. Massage may help.

**Hypertension:** Some women suffer from high blood pressure, especially in the later stages.

**Piles:** As the baby grows, it will push down on the mother's rectum, affecting blood flow.

**Constipation:** Water, fruit, and fiber should get things moving.

**Varicose veins:** Leg veins, especially, tend to swell.

**Cramps:** Stretching and massage relieve the pain.

# Major problems during pregnancy

These conditions are very rare but you need to be aware of the risks. As the saying goes, forewarned is forearmed.

**Gestational diabetes:** A small percentage of mothers develop this condition. Blood-sugar levels can usually be controlled through diet and exercise.

**Low amniotic fluid:** Amniotic fluid is the substance that fills the amniotic sac and supports the baby. If there's too little fluid (a condition known as oligohydramnios) and the mother is nearing full term, labor may be induced.

**Gestational hypertension:** Also called pregnancy-induced hypertension (PIH). This is when the mother develops high blood pressure after 20 weeks of pregnancy. If she develops it late, she may need to be induced or have a C-section. If she develops it early, pre-eclampsia is a risk.

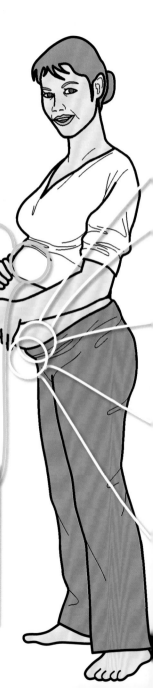

**Premature birth:** Also known as preterm birth, this is when the baby is born before 37 weeks. Around 12 percent of American babies are born prematurely. Some have minor health problems, while others need intensive hospital treatment.

**Placenta previa:** This means the placenta has implanted too low on the wall of the mother's uterus, near the cervix. Early in the pregnancy it rarely causes problems but later on it may cause bleeding and necessitate a C-section delivery.

**Pre-eclampsia:** A combination of high blood pressure and protein in the urine that affects around one in 20 mothers. Untreated, it can develop into eclampsia and life-threatening seizures.

**Miscarriage:** This is when a woman loses the baby during the first 20 weeks of pregnancy. When a miscarriage occurs during the first trimester, the most common cause is problems with the fetus, such as too few or too many chromosomes, or issues with the blood supply to the baby through the placenta.

**C-section (or cesarean):**
See page 42.

# What your pregnant partner can and can't do

Pregnancy takes its toll on a woman's body. Not only is she carrying another human being inside her but, as the fetus grows, it puts pressure on her internal organs.

**Air travel** Flying will not harm the baby but, in the later stages of pregnancy, you don't want to risk your partner going into labor at 30,000 feet. You wouldn't be the first person this has happened to, but it's generally regarded by all involved as a pretty stressful way to bring a child into the world. Some airlines may ask for a doctor's letter confirming your partner is safe to fly. Avoid traveling to countries where vaccinations are required since they can harm the fetus. Pregnant women are more susceptible to blood clots so don't forget the flight socks.

**Exercise** Women who are reasonably fit generally deal with the rigors of childbirth better than women who aren't. However, it's best to keep exercise gentle and low-impact, especially in the later stages. So don't invite your partner for a game of football six months in. Swimming, yoga, and walking are good; any contact sports are not so good. Don't be surprised if she takes up something called pelvic-floor exercises. These strengthen the muscles around the vagina and anus, if you must know, which helps when it comes to childbirth. During pregnancy, these muscles naturally weaken, which can lead to slight incontinence. It's also important to strengthen them after the baby has been born.

**Saunas and Jacuzzis** It's not a great idea to subject the fetus to high temperatures, especially during the first trimester. Your partner should avoid piping hot baths, too. Finnish-style slapping with birch twigs is also off limits. Too bad.

**Sex** Unless there are special medical reasons—and your partner's doctor will make her fully aware of these—it's perfectly healthy to have sex during pregnancy. Bear in mind, though, that you'll be at the mercy of her hormones. In the early stages, morning sickness is likely to put her off the whole idea completely, but by the second trimester, as hormones flood her body, her libido often returns with a vengeance. You may even give her multiple orgasms. Just make sure the positions are comfortable for her. Perhaps ease up on the reverse cowgirl.

During the third trimester, as her body swells to the size of a large rhino, and she feels more tired, the libido is likely to drop again. She will often feel uncomfortable with her body image at this stage. Try reassuring her that she still looks lovely and you might get lucky.

## Morning sickness explained

Early on in the pregnancy, your partner is sure to suffer from morning sickness. Caused by low blood sugar or pregnancy hormones, it can range from mild nausea to full-on vomiting. Some unfortunate women suffer from sickness throughout the entire pregnancy. And ignore the word "morning". It can occur at any time of day.

As the father-to-be, there are certain things you can do to alleviate matters. Become a waiter to your partner. If she wants a ginger infusion and plain piece of toast the minute she wakes up (this is known to help), then leap into action. If she craves high-carbohydrate foods, then oblige her. And bear in mind that her sense of smell will be heightened. Don't come home after a night out, breathing beery fumes all over her.

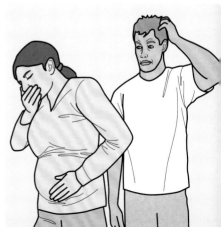

# Foods your partner must avoid

In previous generations, pregnant women seemed to consume just about everything going, including blue cheese, oysters, booze, cigarettes. Nowadays, though, there's a whole list of things that are strictly off limits, either because they harm the baby or because there's a risk of food poisoning.

Since, like a good modern dad, you'll be increasing your culinary contributions in the kitchen, it's a good idea to be aware of what you can and can't put on the menu.

## Avoid:

● Mold-ripened soft cheeses, such as Camembert

● Soft blue cheeses, such as Gorgonzola or Roquefort

● Raw or undercooked eggs

● Unpasteurized milk

● Pâté

● Raw or undercooked meat

● Deli meats

● Liver

● Vitamin A supplements

● Raw shellfish and fish likely to contain high levels of mercury, specifically shark, swordfish, and marlin. Even tuna should be limited

● Fruit or vegetables with soil still clinging to them

● Peanuts

## Cravings explained

Most women get food cravings at some point during their pregnancy, especially in the early stages. These are linked to the increase in hormone levels; and possibly her body is telling her she's low in certain vitamins. Sometimes the cravings get a little out of control, a condition known as pica—women have been found sucking on clay, ashes, or laundry starch—in which case you can help by distracting your partner from what she's craving. Suggest some light outdoor exercise. And hide the coal.

Pregnant women are sometimes repulsed by certain foods they used to love. Coffee and alcohol, in particular, can take on a metallic taste. So while you may still be enjoying the booze, don't be surprised if she goes off it.

# Prenatal and antenatal classes

These vary enormously in style and price, depending on where you live. Whichever classes you choose, do your utmost to go along with your partner. Any advice you can glean will reassure you immensely and allay any fears you might have about the imminent birth. Talking to other expectant dads is particularly useful.

Classes cover areas such as your partner's health, exercises she can do, writing a birth plan, what happens during childbirth, pain relief, postnatal depression, breastfeeding, and basic care of your baby. In the USA, you can attend classes at your hospital or take private classes (the Bradley method or the Lamaze method, for example). In the UK, free classes are available through the NHS and private ones through groups such as the National Childbirth Trust. Hypnobirthing (hypnotherapy during childbirth) is becoming popular all over the western world.

## Prenatal bonding

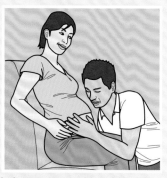

Just because he's still in the womb, it doesn't mean you can't indulge in a spot of bonding with your child. The theory is that fetuses can hear sounds outside the womb from about five months, and that your deeper male voice is more audible than your partner's. Why not gently massage your partner's bump and try to feel the baby moving underneath? Kiss and talk to him through the skin. If you place your ear to your partner's bump, you may even pick out the baby's heartbeat. Try playing soothing music close to the bump. That's Mozart rather than Metallica.

# Birthing options

Your partner may have her heart set on giving birth at home, or you may both agree that you'd prefer to have hospital doctors on hand in case there's an emergency. Perhaps you're registered with a birth center and planning a natural, unmedicated birth. A birthing pool may sound like a good idea. What if she needs an epidural?

Just make sure you both agree on a birth plan well in advance of the big day, and write it down. It's difficult to think straight when her waters have broken and a tiny head is emerging from between her legs. A birth plan will ensure that the midwives know what kind of birth your partner would like, including preferred positions, pain relief, fetal monitoring, and who's going to cut the cord. You both need to be flexible, though. Childbirth rarely goes exactly according to plan.

**Hospitals** Many first-time fathers are understandably apprehensive about choosing a home birth or a birth center, just in case—God forbid!—something goes wrong. It's reassuring to know that the greatest minds and machines in western medicine are on hand if there are any hiccups.

Modern maternity hospitals aren't the soulless, clinical boxes they were when our grandparents were making babies. Some of the more expensive ones make it feel more like a hotel stay. Maternity hospitals have improved massively over the last few decades.

**Birth centers** Many women want their experience of labor to be as natural as possible, but are not quite sure about giving birth at home. In the USA, a birth center can be a happy compromise. These offer a much less clinical environment than a hospital. The mother is either attended to by her OB/GYN or by a midwife and a nurse. In the latter case, a doctor can be summoned from a nearby hospital in an emergency.

Different birth centers offer different facilities. Usually, oxygen and medication are available, as well as baby resuscitation equipment. Mothers are encouraged to give birth drug-free. Visiting family and friends are well catered for. Birth centers are normally less expensive than private hospitals. The British equivalent of a birth center is an NHS midwifery-led unit. Otherwise you could opt for home birth with an NHS midwife in attendance. Similarly, doctors can be called if there's an emergency.

## Hospital versus birth center/home birth

Here are a few factors you should consider when weighing up the pros and cons.

**Access:** Is it easy and quick to get to? Even in rush hour? Parking facilities?

**Security:** You don't want random strangers wandering around.

**Accommodation for dads:** Can you stay the night? Some hospitals (and all birth centers) offer beds to Daddy if Mommy and baby need to stay in overnight.

**Neonatal care:** Different hospitals offer different levels of neonatal care. You may want the extra reassurance that, should a major problem occur, all bases are covered. If you've opted for a birth center, how far away is the nearest maternity hospital?

**Staff:** Are they friendly? What's the nurse-to-patient ratio? In a birth center, are the nurses and midwives all registered?

**Birth records:** Check out the hospital's statistics on number of births, C-sections, and anything else you think relevant.

**Other facilities:** What is the catering like? Are there birthing pools? Is there a mother's labor room in case your partner's labor is drawn out?

**Insurance:** Will you be covered if you start in a birth center and have to transfer to a hospital?

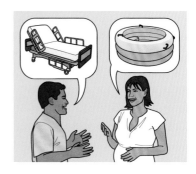

# Get to know your hospital

For some new dads, the first time they see their maternity hospital is after their partner's waters have broken. Big mistake. Make use of any opportunity you can to familiarize yourself with the surroundings into which your baby is going to be born. Many hospitals offer tours of the obstetrical floor so that you can see the labor and birth room (where your baby will enter the world) and the postpartum recovery room (where your partner and baby will recover from the birth). Come the big day, you and your partner don't want to be rubbing shoulders with bleeding gunshot victims because you've stumbled into the wrong ward. Find out exactly where you need to be, what facilities are available, and how it all works. As far as possible, you don't want any hiccups or surprises.

It's crucial to reconnoiter the route from home to hospital well in advance of childbirth. Most American and British hospitals expect you to make your own way there. Are you going to take a taxi? Some drivers will refuse to take a heavily pregnant woman in their vehicle. Are you planning to drive yourself? Surely you're not going to risk public transport? Giving birth on a city bus during rush hour can't be much fun.

# Preparing the nursery

There's a guest coming to stay with you … for at least the next 18 years! Perhaps you have a spare room set aside, or maybe you're going to put him up in your bedroom for the time being. Whatever your options, you need to prepare a special space for your newborn.

Let's assume you have a spare room. Once you're back from the hospital, you'll naturally want your baby to spend his first few weeks of life sleeping in a bassinet next to you. But it's important to establish a disciplined sleep routine early, and that means giving him his own room.

It's not a great idea to subject a newborn to paint fumes, so decorate the room well in advance of the birth. If you already know the sex of your baby, you can make an appropriate color choice. If not, you can always opt for a neutral color scheme. In any case, it will be a fair few years before you have to choose between plastering the room with princess or Star Wars wallpaper.

Have the carpet professionally cleaned and ensure the room is baby- and toddler-safe. Put locks on cupboard doors, and covers over electrical sockets. Get down on the floor and try to put yourself in your baby's shoes, or booties, rather. If there's anything vaguely sharp, you can be sure he will head straight for it the minute he can crawl. See pages 53 and 67 for all the nursery equipment and clothing you will need.

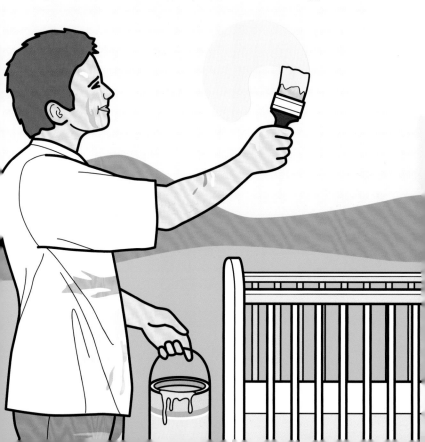

# Dad's pregnant too!

It may sound like the plot of a cheap sci-fi movie, but dads can feel as though they're pregnant. Couvade syndrome is described as a phantom pregnancy that dads-to-be develop in sympathy with their partner's real one. Symptoms include morning sickness, cramps, back pain, mood swings, food cravings, and, in more extreme cases, swollen stomachs that resemble a baby bump. Some dads have even been known to experience labor pains simultaneously with their partner.

While the syndrome is not medically recognized, and may simply be psychosomatic, anecdotal evidence suggests that it might be caused by hormonal changes in the man's body. Just don't hog the toilet when you're throwing up first thing in the morning.

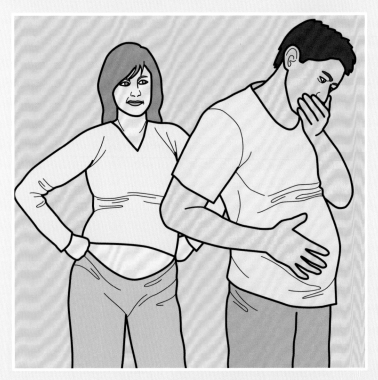

# The sudden birth!

You've seen it in numerous movies. You've probably had the odd nightmare about it. It's rare but it does happen—sometimes labor comes on so quickly that you and your partner don't have time to get to the hospital. Occasionally, a baby can enter the world after just a few pushes. Once you've fought off the initial panic, here's a list of the important things you need to do. It's an unnerving situation to be in, but If you follow these steps, everything should work out fine.

- Call an ambulance.
- Call your doctor and ask him or her to talk you through the process.
- Wash your hands.
- Get lots of clean towels.
- If you value your carpet, put newspapers and old sheets across the floor or the bed where you partner chooses to give birth. Think puppy training.
- When the baby's head is first visible, tell your partner to stop pushing so that her vagina can stretch without tearing.
- As the head emerges, check that the umbilical cord is not around the baby's neck. If it is, use your finger to pull it over his head.
- Catch the baby when he comes out. He will be very slippery. This will be the first of many games of catch that you will play with your child!
- Give the baby to your partner to hold.Place him on her naked chest and dry him off.
- Cover him with a towel.
- Leave the umbilical cord attached.
- If the placenta arrives, put it in a bowl for the doctor or midwife to check later on.
- Admire your baby and wait impatiently for the sound of the ambulance siren.

# PART 2

# THE BIRTH

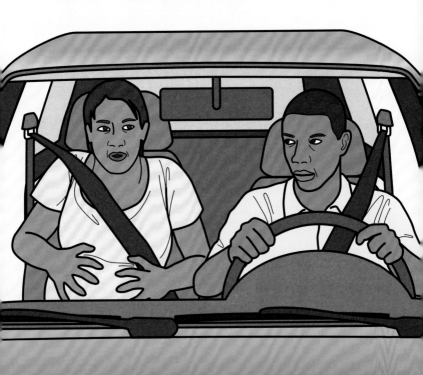

# When to go to hospital

Don't rush to hospital the moment your partner feels the first signs of labor because you'll only be sent back home. Much better to stay in the calm and comfort of your own home until things really start happening. But how do you know when that is?

If her waters break (that is the fluid from the amniotic sac leaking out between her legs), if she's in severe pain, or if she's bleeding, you should head straight for the hospital. Otherwise it's a case of timing the contractions. You can make yourself really useful by operating the stopwatch. Once the contractions are coming regularly, and the time between them is getting shorter, it's normally time to go. Phone the hospital to warn them you're coming. Until then, you'll both be better off at home. She can relax and take her mind off the contractions by reading or watching TV. And you can provide some pain relief and moral support by massaging her back and holding her hand.

It's a good idea to have an overnight bag ready, packed with all your and your partner's essentials. Include all the obvious stuff, such as diapers, baby clothes, blanket, toothbrushes, and pajamas. Don't forget the birth plan (see page 32).

# Is childbirth really that painful?

Here's what comedian Carol Burnett has to say on the subject: "Having a baby is like taking your lower lip and forcing it over your head."

You've got to be realistic. There's going to be some pain, some shouting, some swearing, some tears—a little from you, more from your partner. So while she worries about what's happening inside her body, you should be worrying about the practical things, such as getting her to hospital, getting her to the right part of the hospital, keeping her calm and being her wingman throughout.

# Three stages of labor and birth

The first stage runs from when your partner's contractions begin, up until the point where her cervix is fully dilated. It consists of early labor, when the cervix thins and starts to dilate; active labor, when the dilation of the cervix speeds up, and contractions are stronger, longer, and more frequent; and transition labor, ending in full dilation. It's during active labor that your partner may opt for an epidural. Some women like to walk around during active labor, leaning on something when the contractions come. Encourage her to breathe during the contractions, especially in transition labor.

The second stage runs from full dilation to the birth of your baby. Your partner will now start pushing in order to move the baby down the birth canal. If she wants, you can encourage her verbally. For first-time mothers, this process is normally gradual. The baby's head will appear from between her legs. Some dads find this fascinating and like to see

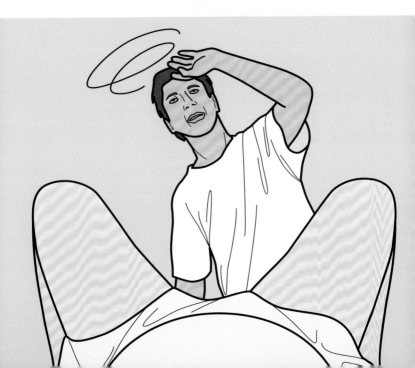

what's going on at the business end. Be warned—it tends to be a bit of a car wreck down there. This woman will become your lover again some day in the near future. Do you really want to see her undercarriage in full childbirth mode? If you're really that interested, why not watch video clips on YouTube? Much less squeamish-making. Don't worry if you start to feel a bit light-headed. There's a lot of blood, and maybe some vomit and poo, too. Just don't pass out. Your partner and the midwives will have quite enough to worry about without you laid flat on the hospital floor.

Finally, your baby will enter the world, helped along by the OB/GYN or the midwife. Provided there are no complications, he will be placed on your partner's chest. Now, once the umbilical cord has been clamped, you'll be asked if you want to cut it. (See Cutting the cord, page 43.)

The third stage lasts from the moment after your partner gives birth until the delivery of the placenta. (See page 44.)

For first-time mothers, labor usually lasts between ten and 20 hours in all, but can be much longer. Best cancel those work meetings.

## Complications

Birth isn't always straightforward. The baby might be breeched, for example, which means he's not in the upside-down position as he should be, but instead has positioned himself feet or backside first. In such circumstances, your partner may need a C-section (very common for first-time mothers, see page 42). In cases where labor is prolonged or there are signs of fetal distress, an assisted delivery may be needed. This is where forceps or vacuum extraction are used to bring your baby out of the birth canal. Forceps delivery involves the gentle use of two tongs to pull out the baby's head. In vacuum extraction, a rounded cup is applied to the baby's head and vacuum pressure used to pull him out. He will often have a raised bruise for a few weeks afterward.

Babies sometimes accidentally ingest meconium (their first poop) which could mean a short hospital stay. Other problems include manual removal of the placenta or vaginal stitching for the mother.

# C-section (or cesarean)

When a normal vaginal birth is dangerous or isn't working, your partner will undergo a C-section.

What with all the blood, it can be a bit unnerving, but it's normally a fairly straightforward process. The surgeon makes a small horizontal incision in the mother's bikini line, then another one in the uterus before lifting the baby out through the resulting hole. "Out of the sunroof" is how some fathers rather flippantly describe it. The amniotic fluid is drained off using suction, the umbilical cord cut, the placenta removed, and the uterus and abdomen stitched back up. Operations usually last between 45 minutes and an hour. The baby is delivered at the beginning, and the rest of the time is spent stitching.

There are two types of C-section—elective and emergency. Elective is when it's planned in advance, usually because of some complication. The anesthetic is normally a spinal rather than a general, which is safer for the baby and allows the mother to hold him as soon as he comes out. A screen is often placed between the mother's head and her abdomen, so she can't see the damage. Unless you're of a particularly hardened nature, you, too, should avoid the business end. The screen can be lowered at the point of delivery—like a magician whipping a rabbit out of a hat.

Emergency C-sections are reserved for when things go awry— perhaps labor fails to progress, or there's a placental hemorrhage, fetal distress, or a prolapsed umbilical cord. An epidural anesthetic will normally be used unless the baby's life is in danger, in which case the mother may be given a general anesthetic.

## Recovery time

Should your partner need a C-section, her body will obviously take a lot longer to recover than if she'd been through straightforward childbirth. Damage from the incisions can take up to six weeks to heal fully. During this time you're going to need to be on hand for simple tasks, such as lifting the baby, housework, and driving the car.

Some women feel disappointment, even despair, after a C-section—they may think they have failed to achieve the perfect birth. If this is the case with your partner, it's worth reminding her that C-section births are far more frequent now than ever before—around a third of American and a quarter of British births are by C-section.

## Cutting the cord

It's easy to feel a bit like a spare part during childbirth. Halfway through, as your partner is sweating and screaming in pain, you may well wonder exactly what you're doing there beside her. So when it comes to cutting the umbilical cord, you can really come into your own. Finally, here's a job that requires the steady hand of the father. And it's a symbolic moment when your child makes the break from the womb into the big wide world.

Experts are divided about when is the best time to cut the cord. There used to be a 30-second rule but in recent years that has been revised. It seems that being attached to the mother for longer allows more blood to be transferred to the baby, reducing iron deficiency.

Take your guidance from the medical staff. She will place two clamps on the cord and give you the go-ahead, showing you exactly where to make the cut (in between the two clamps). Make sure you have a steady hand. Be warned—the cord is tougher than you expect. It's a bit like cutting through a rubber hose. Rest assured, there is no pain for either mother or child.

An umbilical stump, one or two inches long, will remain protruding from his belly button. This will blacken, scab up, and, after ten days or so, fall off. The area must be kept clean and dry at all times, so it doesn't get infected.

## More to come

Once the baby's out, it's not quite all over. There's still the placenta to come. This, the third stage of birth, normally takes place within 15 to 30 minutes of the baby's arrival. It can be a messy affair, as you'd expect when an organ comes out of the mother's womb. She can choose to have a hormone injection which will speed the process up. If your partner has a tear near her vagina from the baby's delivery, it will be sewn up after the placenta comes out.

Many cultures revere the human placenta. Tom Cruise once joked that he planned to eat his baby's placenta. British celebrity chef Hugh Fearnley-Whittingstall really did eat a placenta (fried with shallots and garlic) on TV accompanied by the organ's owner. A word of advice: your friends will soon stop coming round for dinner if placenta's on the menu.

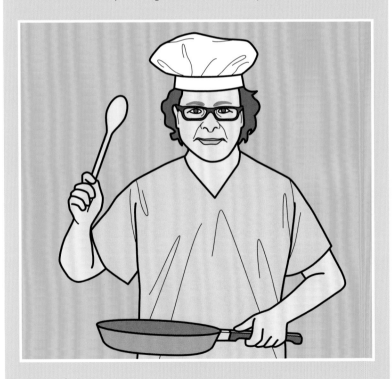

# Meeting your new baby

Welcome to the world! It can be quite a shock the first time a father meets his newborn. This tiny being will be your charge, your offspring, your friend for the rest of your days. It's an important introduction.

Yet not all fathers are immediately captivated by their new babies. Fresh out of the womb, they rarely look their best. E.T., the extraterrestrial, sometimes comes to mind. They are angry-looking with puffy, squinting eyes and covered in a white, waxy substance called vernix. The hospital staff will clean them up, after which the skin goes wrinkly. There may be spots and blotches. Their genitals will look engorged. Their head is often misshapen after its passage through the birth canal. They might be bald or sporting a full head of hair. Some darker babies have hair on their backs and shoulders, even girls. It soon falls off. Most Caucasian babies are born with grayish-blue eyes, while darker races tend to be born with darker eyes. This initial hair color and eye color will change as the baby grows.

Given this description, you can understand why some fathers take time to fall in love with their newborns. Don't worry. You will.

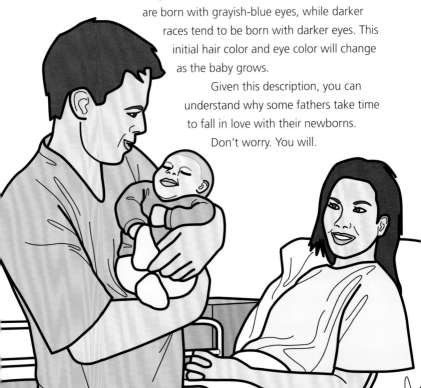

# Naming the baby

You'll spend days, weeks even, discussing, and possibly arguing over, potential baby names with your partner. There's no rush. Many couples, even if they know the sex of the baby in advance, suddenly change their minds once they cast eyes upon their newborn. After all, he might have a huge birthmark on his chest, in which case you can hardly call him Mark; or he might turn out to be a she, putting John-boy out of the question.

Mom and dad rarely agree on a name straightaway, and just wait until the grandparents get involved!

In your favor is the fact that, nowadays, any first name, no matter how unusual it is, seems to be acceptable. If Sylvester Stallone can name his son Sage Moonblood, you can do pretty much whatever you like.

## Worst celebrity baby names

**Nakoa-Wolf Manakauapo Namakaeha**, son of actress Lisa Bonet

**Bronx Mowgli,** son of singer Ashlee Simpson and musician Pete Wentz

**Moxie CrimeFighter,** daughter of magician Penn Jillette

**Pilot Inspektor,** son of actors Jason Lee and Beth Riesgraf

**Moon Unit,** son of singer Frank Zappa

**Kal-El,** son of actor Nicolas Cage

**Audio Science,** son of actress Shannyn Sossamon

**Fifi Trixibelle,** daughter of musician Bob Geldof

**Sage Moonblood,** son of actor Sylvester Stallone

**Jermajesty,** son of singer Jermaine Jackson

**Speck Wildhorse,** son of singer John Mellencamp

**Pirate,** son of singer Jonathan Davis

**Reignbeau,** daughter of actor Ving Rhames

A special mention goes to boxer George Foreman, who named all five of his sons **George** and one of his daughters **Georgetta.**

David Beckham called his son Brooklyn after the neighborhood where he was conceived. Go on, be creative. After all, you don't want him being one of 15 Drakes in his preschool class. Just check the baby's initials don't spell out a rude word.

## Announcing the birth

After 24 hours of labor, the last thing a new mother needs to worry herself with is sending text messages to friends and family on her cell phone. Besides, she'll be too busy swooning over her newborn. That's why it's traditionally the father's role to announce the birth.

In the old days, you'd take out an announcement in the newspapers. Thanks to modern technology, you can now alert friends and family a lot quicker than that. It's important to break the good news to those nearest and dearest to you first. Your Mom and Dad, and your partner's parents, will be very upset if the first they hear about their grandchild is via Facebook and not directly from you. So call the people closest to you on the phone and tell them as soon as you can.

After that, you might want to text-message everyone else. Better still, take a photo of your pride and joy, and send out a group email. Include information such as the time of birth, the baby's weight (people who have had kids love to know this, whereas childless men often don't understand the relevance), the mother's physical well-being, and, of course, the baby's name, if you've already chosen it.

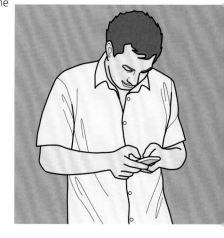

Soon enough you'll be back home on your social media networks and announcing this major event in your life to the entire world.

# On show

Relatives, especially the two grandmothers, will be champing at the bit to meet the latest addition to the family. If childbirth has been relatively straightforward, this shouldn't pose any problems. As new parents, you and your partner will probably be proud to show off the little human being you have created, so invite close friends and family to coo over Junior.

Just bear in mind how exhausted your partner will be. She may have just limped across the finish line after a marathon birthing ordeal. And she won't be looking her best. The last thing she needs is an overbearing father-in-law zooming in with his iPhone.

Visitors will naturally ask to cuddle the newborn. Ask them to wash their hands first to reduce risk of infection. If the mother has been operated on she may not be able to receive visitors immediately.

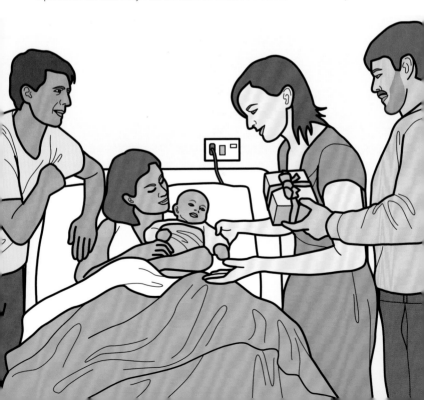

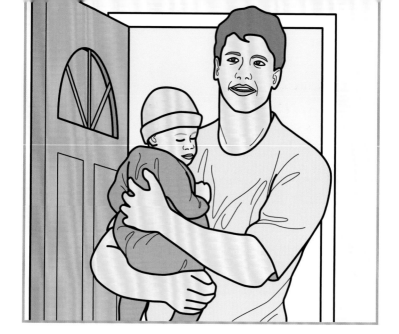

## Taking baby home

American and British hospitals won't allow you to drive your new baby home unless you have a proper child car seat. (See Baby transport, page 80.) Never strap a child seat onto the front seat in case the airbags inflate.

## Birth defects

Better not to dwell on this, but bear in mind that birth defects are a possibility. (Mostly, you will know about serious birth defects in advance.) Medical staff check for them once the baby is born. Rare possibilities include Down's syndrome, spina bifida (spinal vertebrae do not fuse properly), cerebral palsy (muscular paralysis), club foot, cleft lips, cleft palates, and dislocation of the hip. Thankfully, modern medicine can effectively treat many of them. The best thing you can do if such a scenario arises is to support your partner and child as best you can.

# PART 3

# BABY CARE

## Paternity leave

In days gone by, new dads might have taken just the afternoon off work to toast their newborn. Nowadays they have statutory rights so that they can properly bond with their baby.

In the USA, the Family and Medical Leave Act of 1993 grants employees up to 12 weeks of unpaid leave. In the UK, new dads are entitled to at least two weeks' paid paternity leave. At the time of publication, the statutory amount was just over £135 per week.

Various bureaucratic rules govern paternity leave in both countries but most employers are pretty flexible. You obviously can't predict the exact date of the birth. Aim to take the bulk of your leave after your little one arrives.

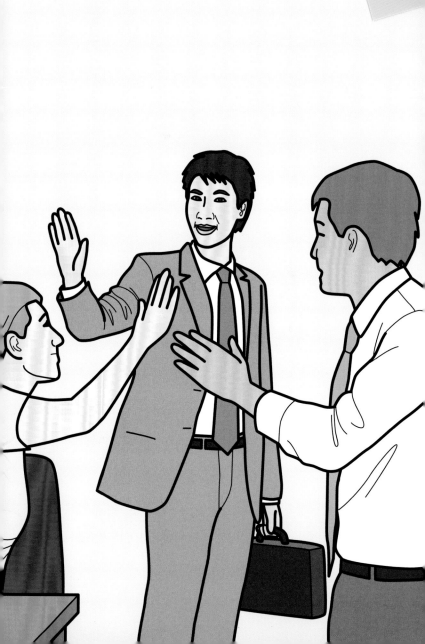

# Wet the baby's head

After the stress of childbirth, you're going to be in dire need of a drink. Just as well, then, that it's a tradition for the father to invite all his friends for a few drinks to celebrate his new role as Daddy. It's called wetting the baby's head.

In the old days, it was just male friends who would crack open the Champagne, but nowadays you might invite all your and your partner's friends at the same time. And what better excuse to enjoy those Cuban cigars you've been saving?

Depending on your religion (or lack thereof), you might be planning a christening or brit milah. This is another chance for you to show off the little one to all your friends and family, and to appoint godparents. Don't be surprised if your male friends are fairly underwhelmed with the new addition to the family. Babies do all look pretty much the same.

# Your new tenant

The day you take your new baby home, you'll be so excited that adrenalin will be coursing through your veins. Not everyone will share that excitement. Older kids, step-kids, and pets might not initially warm to the new arrival. Expect some jealousy. It's a good idea to buy a gift for any older kids and tell them it's from the baby. Over the first few days, encourage them to take an interest in the newborn.

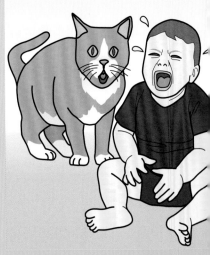

If the baby is your first, pets can pose problems, too. They may see him as an intruder. One way to get around this situation is to introduce the pet to the baby's scent before you bring him home from the hospital. Perhaps give the pet one of the baby's blankets so that it can familiarize itself with your baby's smell. Never leave pets, even the gentlest ones, alone with newborns. All animals take a while to get used to new family members.

# Nursery furniture

Now for the crib. Good luck when it comes to assembling it. We may have flown men to the moon but we still haven't designed a baby crib that's easy to put together. Set aside several hours for this particular task.

Place the crib away from windows, direct sunlight, lamps, radiators, and air-conditioners. Get a mesh crib bumper—the band that stretches around the bottom of the crib, inside it. The quilted types have been known to cause accidental suffocation.

You'll need a changing station, too, although if you haven't the space for one, you can change the baby's diapers on a changing mat on the floor. A proper changing table features a top level, where you lay your baby, and a shelf below, where you put all the diaper-changing paraphernalia, and there's a lot more than you'd ever expect (see page 64).

## Nursery equipment checklist

- Bassinet/Moses basket
- Crib and mattress
- Fitted sheets
- Swaddling blankets
- Baby monitor
- Sealed diaper bin
- Changing table
- Diapers (thousands of them!)
- Baby wipes (cotton wool and warm water for newborns)
- Comfortable chair for breastfeeding

## Which baby monitor?

While your partner takes care of the baby developing inside her, when it comes to choosing a baby monitor, you can make yourself useful.

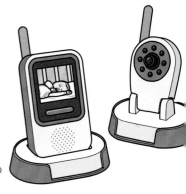

Dozens of models are available, ranging from simple walkie-talkies to full-on digital video monitors that link to your smartphone. Do you really need to watch your little one sleeping in high-definition video, though? Do you honestly plan to sit around the dining table watching him sleep? Why not go for a simpler model and spend the money you save on an upmarket stroller? Just make sure the monitor's range will cover your entire house and backyard. Unfortunately, they're unlikely to stretch as far as the local drinking hole.

## Movement monitors

In recent years, parents have become much more aware of the risks of SIDS (sudden infant death syndrome, or cot death). You can now buy movement monitors, which are fixed beneath the baby's mattress, or on his clothing, and set off an alarm should he stop moving for a certain period of time—reassuring if you're a nervous parent, but perhaps a bit excessive.

# Breastfeeding

Sorry, buddy. As much as you want to be a modern dad and help whenever you can, this is one area where, for obvious anatomical reasons, you will always be utterly useless.

However, you can offer your partner lots of moral support. Natural breastfeeding isn't always straightforward—the baby will usually take a while to get the hang of it; the milk flow isn't always regular; mother can get very sore nipples, clogged milk ducts, or even mastitis (an infection in the breasts).

Breastfeeding mothers become extremely thirsty as the fluids in their body are passed on to the baby, so always be on hand with a glass or two of drinking water for your partner. There will be regular feeds throughout the day, around six to eight of them for a newborn baby, which, after the novelty has worn off, can be mind-numbingly boring for the mother. Help her by setting up a comfortable feeding chair and arranging a good position for watching television. A TV in the bedroom will help pass the time during night feeds. As the baby grows, the number of feeds will drop—to around two or three a day by the time he's six months old.

## Breastfeeding in public

Attitudes to public breastfeeding differ enormously across the western world. Big cities tend to be more liberal, so that if your partner started breastfeeding in a restaurant in New York or London, passers-by would barely bat an eyelid. Do the same thing in a small hick town and you may empty the room—good riddance. Always remember that your partner is entirely within her right to breastfeed wherever she likes. It is legal all across the UK and, as of July 2018, in all 50 states of the USA. Having the law on your side doesn't necessarily make it easy when a narrow-minded conservative starts tutting and passing comment. He or she is in the wrong and should be ignored.

It can take time for your partner to become comfortable baring her breasts in public. Be there to support her, perhaps by offering a muslin or blanket to cover up the baby. To build up confidence suggest attempting the first few feeds in a quiet café, rather than on a busy commuter train. It should soon become second nature.

# Bottle-feeding

Mommy can't be around every moment of every day. She'll need the odd break from her baby, otherwise she'll go insane. She may even have decided to go back to work. This doesn't mean breast milk needs to stop entirely. Many women choose to express milk using a breast pump, and then store it in the refrigerator or freezer.

Although experts disagree on storage time, the general advice is that breast milk will last up to a week in the refrigerator and up to six months in the freezer. Use sterilized bottles for the fridge and specially designed freezer bags when it's going on ice. Don't worry if the milk separates after it's been in the fridge for a while—simply give it a shake before you pop it in Junior's mouth.

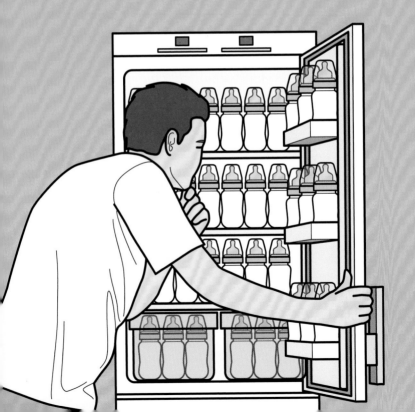

After nine months of pregnancy, there's a good chance your partner will be dying for a proper drink. She may even—God forbid!—be invited to a party. As long as she's expressed enough milk in advance, there's no reason why she shouldn't enjoy a small amount of alcohol. When you get home, you can give the baby the expressed milk while her body naturally washes away any booze she may have consumed. Otherwise she can do a "pump and dump"—she pumps out the milk in her body that has alcohol in it and throws it away. (Don't tell the doctors. Those killjoys will ban any alcohol from a breastfeeding woman. Just don't let her overdo it!)

When bottle-feeding starts, a new father suddenly comes into his own. Once a breastfeeding routine has been established, you may want to introduce the odd bottle of expressed milk, just to get your baby used to another way of feeding. It can take a while for him to take to the bottle, however.

**Preparing bottles** Milk bottles and nipples (teats) need to be meticulously sterilized before each use for at least the first year of your baby's life. Start off by washing them thoroughly, using dishwashing liquid and a special bottle brush, or put them in the dishwasher on a hot wash. Be sure to remove any milk residue from all surfaces of the bottles, caps, and nipples. Nipples can be turned inside out so the inside can be thoroughly cleaned.

Now comes the boiling part. Yes, you can use the old-fashioned method by boiling the bottles and parts for ten minutes or so in a saucepan. But let's be realistic—you haven't got time for all that ass-ache. You're going to be doing this chore at least twice a day and you need to get it done quickly. Opt instead for a microwave or electric sterilization system. There are various brands on the market. Microwave systems involve placing the bottles inside a plastic case, which then fits inside your microwave. Electric versions are separate machines that you plug into the power supply and in which you place all the bottles. If space is at a premium in your kitchen, choose the microwave version.

**Formula milk** Up until the first time you are asked to buy some for your child, you will probably think all baby milk is pretty much the same. Wrong! Walk down the baby aisle of any supermarket in the western world and you'll be dazzled by the huge array of different baby milk formulas available. Mostly derived from cow's milk, these are separated into different groups depending on the age of your baby. Try to stick to the same brand so his digestive system gets used to it. Some scientists are concerned that soya-milk formula contains high levels of estrogen and may weaken a baby's immune system.

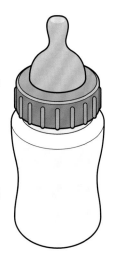

Formula milk normally comes in powder form. Making a batch is an easy enough process—a feed is made up by mixing it with cold water that has been previously boiled. It is important that you follow the instructions and portions given on the packet to the letter. Too much water and your baby won't get the required nourishment; too much powder and he risks dehydration or constipation. Neither of these outcomes results in a very happy child, so make the sensible choice and do what the label tells you to.

Babies won't always drink the same amount at each feed. If he sinks the entire contents of the bottle like a thirsty alcoholic, you can make up another bottle and offer him some more. On the other hand, if he stops sucking and rejects the bottle, perhaps he's had enough and there's no need to try to force the issue.

**Heating the milk** Babies prefer milk at body temperature. Unfortunately, the microwave is no good since it heats milk unevenly and pockets of very hot milk could scald the baby's mouth. Instead, place the bottle in a container of recently boiled water. After a couple of minutes, swirl it around and squirt a bit onto your wrist to test the milk is at the right temperature.

When you're away from home, it can be difficult to warm up a bottle of milk. Either warm it before you head out and keep it in an insulated bottle bag, or call into the nearest café at feed time and ask them to heat it for you. Some café owners get a little precious about milk-warming, worried they might get sued should the baby be scalded. To avoid this, ask for a bowl of boiling water rather than use of their microwave. At a push, bottles can be warmed up under your armpit or down your pants.

**Holding the bottle** At home, prepare yourself and your baby by sitting comfortably in your favorite armchair with your favorite TV show

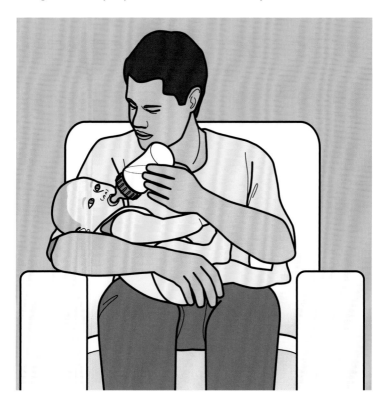

cued up and ready to play. Hold the baby in a cradle position in your non-dominant arm, with his head raised above his tummy and supported by the crook of your elbow. Then use your dominant hand to feed him the bottle.

Once he's used to sucking on a bottle nipple, he'll latch on quickly. Your main concern should be that he swallows milk but no air, otherwise you risk giving him painful indigestion or making him sick. Experience fresh baby vomit down your front just once and you'll instantly realize this is not a good idea. For that reason, you need to make sure there are no air bubbles in the teat before you place it in his mouth. From then on, keep the bottle at a 45-degree angle, however vigorously he's sucking on it, so that no air bubbles get into the milk.

If he wants to, let your baby rest halfway through the feed. Use this interval to burp him.

**Baby burping** As he gobbles down the milk, you'll notice that your baby's tummy will start to get bigger and bigger. While the sight of your baby turning into a miniature buddha may amuse you, wind will inevitably get trapped in the stomach and, if you want something resembling a decent night's sleep, you need to release it. Place a burping cloth (or muslin, as the British call it) over your shoulder to protect your clothes. Vomit stains down the back of your shirt are never a particularly good look. Hold the baby against you with his tummy next to your chest, his head over your shoulder, and your dominant hand under his bottom. Use your other hand to pat his back gently, or make circular motions with your hand until he burps. Be patient—this can take quite a long time. To try to speed things up, bouncing the baby very lightly will help the air pass through his system.

You can also sit him on your lap and rub his back, or lay him face down across your lap. Just make sure his head doesn't drop below his tummy, or else it's baby-puke time.

## Pacifier or no pacifier?

Love 'em or loathe 'em, pacifiers (or dummies, as they're known in the UK) are a quick and easy way to turn off baby tears. Trouble is, babies easily get hooked on them. Before going down the pacifier route, consider the following drawbacks.

- Early use of a pacifier can cause problems with breastfeeding because the baby confuses the rubber teat with the human one.
- If a pacifier falls out of the baby's mouth at night, he will often wake up in distress.
- Pacifiers can delay speech development because babies suck on them when they could be practicing speaking.
- The constant presence of a pacifier in the mouth can cause protruding teeth later in life.
- Sucking a pacifier becomes an addictive habit that's hard to break and could last for years to come in the form of thumb sucking.

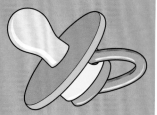

## Hiring a maternity nurse (or doula)

They're expensive, but that's because they make life so much easier for new parents. Maternity nurses will help during those turbulent first few weeks with issues such as breastfeeding, diaper-changing, sleeping patterns, and baby routines. They stay with you in your home so as to be on hand at all times. You should seriously consider hiring one if your partner's undergone a C-section or if you have a hectic work schedule and can't take paternity leave. It may help keep your partner sane. Needless to say, maternity nurses must be professional and registered.

# Bathing the baby

This can be a really fun job for a new dad. During the initial period of fatherhood, you might sometimes feel a little removed from the action, but giving your baby a bath provides the perfect opportunity for a bit of bonding time together. For the first few weeks of his life, provided you keep him clean during diaper changes, you only need to give him what's known as a "top and tail bath" a couple of times a week. Lay him on a towel and use pieces of absorbent cotton wool dipped in cooled (but already boiled) water. He shouldn't be placed in a proper bathtub until his umbilical stump has healed and dropped off.

From then on, given the enormous amounts of poop he will generate, you'll want to bath him once a day—more if the poop gets particularly messy. It's not unknown for a spectacularly enthusiastic delivery to project all the way up his back. Before bed is the perfect bathtime, since the warm water will relax him and, you hope, make him feel sleepy.

Most dads and babies (once they get used to the sensation) love bathtime. He will enjoy the feeling of splashing around in water and you will love the chance to bond with him. Be warned, though—do not leave the bathroom for even a second. He may have spent nine months in the womb but, now he's out in the big wide world, he can no longer breathe underwater. Babies can't turn themselves over and may drown in just a few inches of water.

You can bath him in your own bathtub if you like (just make sure you keep the water shallow) but baby bathtubs (specially shaped plastic containers) will offer support for his head and give you an extra hand to wash him with. Make sure the bathroom is warm and the water is comfortable. If you are really keen, you can check the water temperature with a baby thermometer. This isn't really necessary—you can feel the temperature perfectly well with your wrist.

Place your baby in the bathtub, cupping his head under one hand. Using pieces of absorbent cotton wool and baby soap—choose from among the countless products available—wash his face first, then the rest of his body, ending up around the diaper area where, inevitably, he will be grubbiest. Don't wash underneath the foreskin—there's no need. With baby girls, wash the vagina first, wiping back toward the bottom. Finish by rinsing off any excess soap with water.

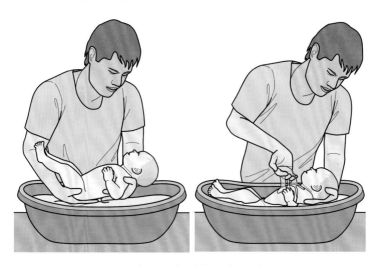

Once or twice a week, you should gently wash your baby's scalp using baby shampoo. Many newborns develop something called cradle cap, a crusty skin rash that appears on the scalp. It's painless and perfectly normal.

Now take the baby out of the tub and wrap him in a clean towel, dabbing him dry. Before you dress him for bed, you can let him wriggle on the towel. The more you can allow air to reach his naked bottom, the less likely he is to get diaper rash.

# Poop alert!

Don't for a minute think you can avoid poop. It's a fact of life that babies are crap-making machines. For the first six months of their lives, it's all they live for. That and vomiting. Newborns can need ten or more diaper changes in a single day, especially if they're breastfeeding, so get used to it. Become an expert at diaper changing. Hold your nose and embrace the poop.

What will surprise you initially is the color. The first poo a baby delivers is greenish-black and sticky, like tar. Called meconium, it contains amniotic fluid, bile, mucus, and the like, which collects in his tummy while he's in the womb.

From then on, you can expect various hues of poop, ranging from mustard-yellow, if he's breastfeeding, to sandy-colored, if he's on formula milk, and even the dreaded green stuff. Sometimes you can be forgiven for suspecting a duck has crapped all over your living-room carpet, not a tiny, lovely human being.

Make sure you change messy diapers promptly, otherwise you risk the dreaded diaper rash, not to mention a less-than-fragrant household.

## Boys versus girls

Poop is poop whether it comes out of a baby girl or a baby boy. However, the method of cleaning up said substance differs according to gender.

**Changing a baby boy's diaper** Watch out for the projectile peeing! You'll be mid-diaper change, confident that everything is going swimmingly when, suddenly, a jet of urine will splash in your face. It will only happen the once. After that, you'll always remember to keep his penis covered with a piece of tissue. It's perfectly normal for baby boys to get an erection during a diaper change. Dads should be proud it all works correctly.

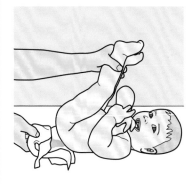

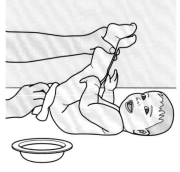

**1** To start off, unfasten the diaper and survey the damage. Use the soiled diaper to wipe away the lion's share and then be meticulous about mopping up any poo that remains.

**2** For babies under a month old, use cotton balls and lukewarm water; otherwise it's baby wipes. There's a good chance that poo will leak all over your baby's clothes before you notice he needs changing. So have a change of clothes ready (for him and, in dire cases, for you as well).

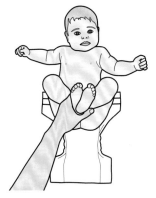

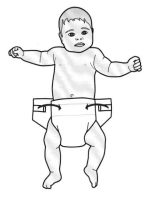

**3** Lift the baby's legs and place the reverse of the clean diaper under his back, with the fastening tabs out to the side. Keep his penis pointing down otherwise he'll soak his clothes when he later wees.

**4** Then fold the front of the diaper up through his raised legs onto his belly and bring the tabs in from the sides, pressing them firmly onto his tummy. The fit should be snug, but not too tight.

**Changing a baby girl's diaper** With a baby girl you may not get the projectile peeing problem, but you must bear in mind that poo can get into the vagina area. Remove it all with thorough wiping, moving from front to back to avoid infection.

## Avoiding diaper rash

All babies will suffer from diaper rash in varying degrees, especially around the bottom. You can keep it to a minimum by applying a barrier cream—zinc oxide- or petroleum-jelly-based—or a diaper-rash cream. Loads of brands are available. Desitin is popular in the US, while Sudocrem is a favorite in the UK.

Once you've cleaned and dried your baby thoroughly, lay him naked from the waist down on a towel for as long as you can, to allow fresh air to the skin. Then apply the cream and put on the diaper.

## Washable or disposable diapers?

The jury is out on whether washable diapers really are that much more eco-friendly than disposable ones. Once you factor in the extra energy you use washing and drying reusable diapers, you realize that both methods have a heavy carbon footprint. True, it's horrendous how many disposable diapers your baby goes through. All of it ends up in landfill. But any environmental concerns you have will quickly evaporate once you're knee deep in poop. Disposable diapers are much easier and less time-consuming. Worry about the planet once he's learned to control his bowels.

## Table or mat

Diaper-changing stations are two-tiered tables with a changing mat on top and all the diaper paraphernalia stored underneath. What with all the other baby equipment, you may not have room for a table, especially if the baby is sharing your bedroom. In that case, use a changing mat on the floor—no risk, then, that the baby might fall off.

# Baby clothes

Before long, you'll find yourself drowning in your baby's clothes. The laundry basket will overflow with dirty garments. The washing machine will take a severe battering. Where do all these clothes come from? While your partner will no doubt have sensibly stocked up, a lot of them will be gifts from friends and family. And just as well, since you won't believe how quickly you get through them.

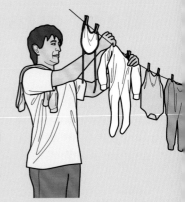

## Clothing checklist

So what are the essential items you need in your life? Here's a list.

- **One-piece outfits:** Also known as babygros or onesies, these all-in-one suits are for both daytime and nighttime wear, and cover a baby from neck to toe. Go for poppers, not buttons. The latter will drive you insane.

- **One-piece shirts:** A T-shirt that fastens underneath the baby's crotch, allowing easy access to a nasty diaper.

- **Socks:** These get kicked off constantly and left in the park, so stock up.

- **Booties:** Soft shoes, moccasin-style, so easy to get on and off.

- **Scratch mittens:** Essential when he's really young to stop him scratching his face with his fingernails. Some one-piece outfits have mittens built in.

- **Cardigan sweaters:** As many as you like, all with the obligatory cute animal embroidered on them.

- **Hats:** No, not a Mets baseball cap. Baby hats need to be made of cotton and close-fitting.

- **Sunhats:** To prevent his bald head from getting burned in the summer sunshine.

- **Snowsuits:** For those outdoor winter expeditions.

- **Bibs:** For vomit and other treats

- **Burping cloths (muslins):** Ditto.

# Baby ailments

They're tiny, they're helpless, and their immune systems and organs haven't fully developed. No wonder many newborns suffer from the occasional medical issue. Dads should be able to spot what's going on and help alleviate the problem. If you're at all worried, contact your doctor. Breastfed babies are normally protected from more serious diseases by antibodies in their mother's milk.

**Colic:** Long-term indigestion and excessive crying that affects baby boys more than girls. Massaging his tummy may help. Baby medicines, such as Infacol, are available.

**Anaphylactic shock:**
A severe allergic reaction caused by nuts, shellfish, insect bites, or stings. Symptoms include swelling, breathing problems, hives, vomiting, and diarrhea. Call for paramedics who will probably inject him with epinephrine.

**Croup:** A deep, hoarse cough like an angry seal's. It's caused by a swelling of the baby's throat and voice box, and should pass within a week or so.

**Diaper rash:** See page 66.

**Diarrhea:** Viruses, bacteria, food allergies, and too much juice are among the many reasons your baby might come down with the runs. The important thing is to keep him hydrated. If he's not also throwing up, give him milk. Otherwise, you can get a pediatric electrolyte solution from the drugstore or pharmacy.

**Eczema:** An itchy skin rash, especially around the wrists, the backs of the knees, and the insides of the elbows. Many babies suffer from it. Using soap-free body wash helps, as does emollient skin cream.

**Whooping cough:** Cold-like symptoms that develop into a very serious cough, caused by bacteria that inflame the baby's lungs and airways. Coughing spells can sometimes last up to 30 seconds. It's important to consult a doctor, who will probably give the baby antibiotics (and you a very welcome pair of earplugs).

**Fever:** A high body temperature (see below) is usually a sign of fever. Doctors may suggest children's acetaminophen (Tylenol or paracetamol) or ibuprofen and Advil (if he's six months or older).

# Taking temperature

Ideally, your baby's body temperature should be 97.7 to 99.5°F (36.5 to 37.5°C), slightly higher than an adult's. This will vary slightly throughout the day—lower in the morning and higher in the evening.

First, you need to decide what kind of thermometer to want to buy. There are digital models that you roll across his forehead, and others that you stick in his ear, his mouth, under his arm, or even up his bottom. How much are you prepared to spend? Which orifice are you planning to put it in?!

Forehead and underarm thermometers are the least accurate, rectal ones the most accurate. Oral thermometers are tricky to use because babies find the sensation uncomfortable.

Before inserting a rectal thermometer, lubricate it with petroleum jelly. Place your baby face down on a mat, spread his buttocks slightly, and gently insert the thermometer (but no more than one inch). Keep a firm grip on his buttocks so that the thermometer stays in until it bleeps. Don't be shocked if he poops after the thermometer is removed. (You probably would, too!)

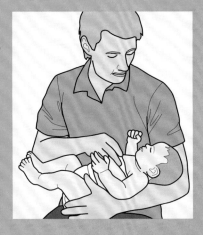

Avoid taking your baby's temperature immediately after a bath when he will be warmer than normal.

## Spotting meningitis

All parents should look out for signs of meningitis. Thankfully, it's rare but early diagnosis is crucial since it attacks the brain or spinal cord and, in extreme cases, can kill a baby. Don't take any unnecessary chances; if you are concerned head for hospital at the first signs.

Symptoms can start off looking very similar to those of flu or a bad cold. Others to look out for include:

- Irritability and refusal of food
- Floppiness, unresponsiveness, or stiffness with jerking movements
- High-pitched crying or moaning
- Pale, blotchy skin
- Vomiting
- Sleepiness
- A swollen fontanel (the soft part on top of the head)
- Sensitivity to light

# How to hold the baby

Unless you were quite a bit older than your siblings when they were born or have nieces or nephews, it's actually surprisingly easy to get pretty far through life without ever holding a baby.

Newborns tend to be fairly floppy, like rubber chickens—except, unlike rubber chickens, you can't throw them around the room. You need to learn how to hold them properly. Remember that newborns don't have the neck muscles to hold their heads up.

**Baby pick-up** When the baby is lying down, slide your dominant hand under his head and neck, and your other hand under his bottom and spine.

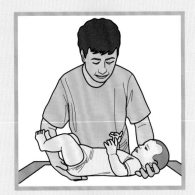

**Cradle hold** With your right hand under his head and neck, and your left hand under his bottom and spine, place the baby against your chest. His right ear will be close to your heartbeat, which will reassure him and possibly send him to sleep.

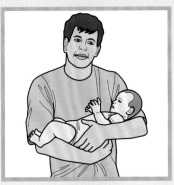

**Shoulder hold** Use your non-dominant hand to support his head and neck. Placing your dominant hand under his bottom, lift him up so his head rests on your shoulder. This is the perfect position for him just after he's had his milk, although beware of potential sick down your back. Wise dads tend to cover their shoulders with a burping cloth.

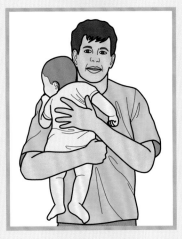

# Time for bed

Most parents put their newborn to sleep in a bassinet (called a Moses basket in the UK) or crib next to their bed for the first few weeks of his life. It's reassuring to have him sleeping so close and it makes breastfeeding during the night a lot easier. But some babies are restless or noisy sleepers. The sooner you can get him used to sleeping in his own room, with a regular routine, the better.

Research has proven that babies who sleep on their backs with their feet right down at the base of the crib are less prone to SIDS (see page 74), so all the experts now recommend this position.

It's important to keep your baby calm before bedtime. Turn the lights low, keep your voice to a whisper, and don't play any games. He will soon learn these are the signals for sleepy time. Gentle rocking,

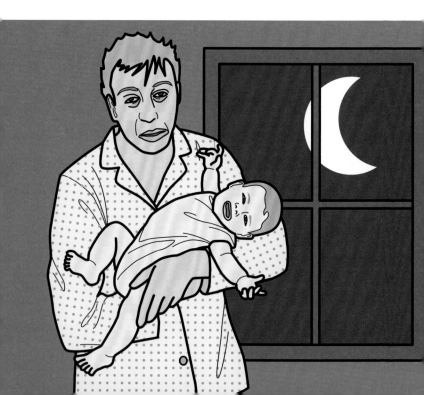

cuddling, or lullabies will add to the soporific effect (for both you and him). Don't be surprised if you wake up an hour later, drooling on the floor of his nursery.

Total sleeping time obviously differs from baby to baby, just as it does from adult to adult. As a general rule, a newborn will sleep for around 16 hours a day, while a one-year-old will manage about 14 hours a day. If only it was all at once. Imagine how easy parenting would be. Sadly, he will take his sleep in two to four-hour blocks, which means you and your partner will have to follow suit. Ever wondered why new parents always have bags under their eyes? You have to face the fact that, during the early months, you and your partner are going to be up several times during the night, feeding, changing, and comforting him.

After six or eight weeks, things will start to improve. His daytime sleeps will get shorter and his nighttime sleeps will (hopefully) get longer. He may even start to sleep through the night—the ultimate prize for every new parent. This may not be the case with your little one, though. Some toddlers still wake up every night.

## How to establish good sleep routines

Don't let him get overtired. Bizarrely, this will make it harder for him to fall asleep. Respond to signs that he may be tired, such as crying and rubbing his eyes.

**Blackout blinds:** They will help with daytime naps.

**Night versus day**: Interact with him during the day so he associates daylight with being awake. If he wakes during the night, keep the lights low and sound to a minimum.

**Bedtime routines:** Baths, lullabies, and stories will all help to teach him that now is the time to go to sleep.

**Set the times:** Put him to bed at night and for naps at the same time every day. This will help train his body clock.

## Bedtime stories

While there's little point in reading *Harry Potter* stories to a newborn, once he's a few months old he will start responding to baby books. Some excellent touch-and-feel books are available, and ones with noisy buttons to press. It's good to establish a bedtime story routine early on in his life so that he's comfortable with books once he starts learning to read.

## The danger of SIDS (cot death)

The very thought of sudden infant death syndrome can keep new parents awake at night, sick with worry—and not surprisingly. More than 2,000 babies in the USA and 300 in the UK die every year because of SIDS. Medical experts aren't sure of the exact cause—there are probably several causes. Fret not, however. It's still a rare occurrence, and there are several ways in which you can reduce the risk:

● Swaddle your baby and have him sleep on his back with his feet at the base of the crib.

● Breastfeed your baby.

● Apply a no-smoking rule in the house.

● Keep his room ventilated and not too warm.

● Don't overdress your baby.

● Avoid very soft mattresses, excess bedding, and stuffed toys in his crib.

## Swaddling

At first, it will feel strange to truss your baby up like a parcel, but he'll get a much better night's sleep if you swaddle him. It will keep him warm and secure, a bit like he was in the womb, and stop him waking himself up with his flailing limbs. (Yes, babies do tend to flail their limbs.)

Be sure to leave enough room at the bottom of the swaddling blanket so that he can move his legs up and away from his body. Wrap it too tightly and you risk damaging the cartilage in his hip sockets, possibly leading to hip dysplasia (dislocation of the hip.) As your baby reaches six or eight weeks old, he will let you know by kicking or crying that swaddling is no longer his thing.

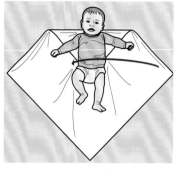

**1** Place a large blanket flat on your bed in a diamond shape. Fold the top point of the diamond down around 6in. (15cm) so that you have a straight edge, and place the baby on the blanket with his head just protruding over the top of this straight edge.

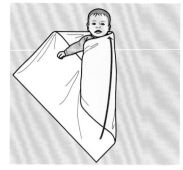

**2** Draw the right-side point (as you're looking at it) of the diamond over your baby's body and arm and tuck it beneath the other arm and behind his back.

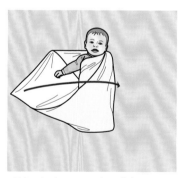

**3** Take the bottom point of the diamond and draw it over his left shoulder. Make sure you leave enough room at the bottom of the blanket so he can move his legs up and away from his body.

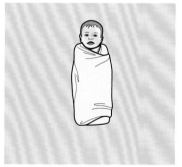

**4** Draw the remaining point of the diamond across his body and tuck it behind his back. He should be wrapped securely but not so tightly that he's uncomfortable.

# Baby meltdowns

All babies have meltdowns. Some last for minutes, while others seem to go on all day until you're ready to tear your hair out. Remember that crying is how babies communicate.

There could be any number of reasons he's grumpy—he's hungry, he's tired, he's ill, he's hot, he's cold, he's bored, he wants to be cuddled, he's got wind, he's teething, you've accidentally stepped on his finger. Once you've checked for all the obvious problems, you may find the crying still carries on regardless. What you need are some distraction tricks.

**Something to suck:** Pacifiers really do work. (See the pros and cons, though, page 61.) Even your finger will soothe him.

**Music:** Lullabies work better than Foo Fighters (although start a baby young on good rock 'n' roll!).

**Fresh air:** A walk around the backyard may be just what he needs to calm down.

**Swaddling:** See page 74.

**Rocking:** Cradle him back and forth in your arms, or put him in a bouncy seat—both work well.

**Massage:** Use some olive oil and keep it gentle.

**Drive in the car:** The motion and change of scenery often lull him to sleep.

While all this is going on, there's no point in both you and your partner listening to your baby crying incessantly. Take it in turns to take a break, otherwise you'll both end up going insane. A few moments' peace will make the situation much more bearable.

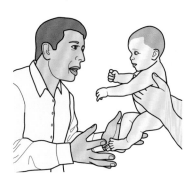

## Baby decibels

Ever wondered just how loud that crying can get? Some babies have had their screams measured as high as 130 decibels, around the same as a Metallica concert or a power mower. Why not invest in a pair of ear defenders? After all, the law says you shouldn't be subjected to that kind of noise in the workplace.

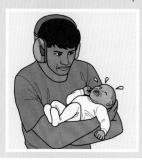

## Tough love

When babies really won't stop crying whatever you do, and you're both on your knees with exhaustion, it's time to consider some tough love. It's time to ignore the crying. Experts don't recommend this until the baby is at least four or five months old. It can be very tough to stick it out, since the first time you do it your baby may continue crying for 30 minutes before falling asleep. The theory is as he learns that you won't run to him every time he complains, the length of crying shortens. Be sure to check for all the usual problems first, though.

# Baby immunizations up to one year

Official recommendations for baby immunizations are changing all the time, so check with your doctor or midwife for the latest advice. Here is a very general guide to shots he will need up to the age of one year (official US and UK NHS recommendations at the time of printing). Some immunizations continue after the age of one.

The first time you willingly offer up your baby for injection, it will break your heart. He's so tiny and that needle's so big! But by the time he's gone for his fifth shot, you'll be pretty blasé about the whole thing.

**US Recommended Immunization Schedule:**
**Birth:** Hepatitis B
**One to two months:** Hepatitis B
**Two months:** DTaP (diptheria, tetanus, and pertussis, or whooping cough), Hib (hemophilus influenza type B), IPV (polio), PCV (pneumococcal disease), Rotavirus
**Four months:** DTaP, Hib, IPV, PCV, Rotavirus
**Six months:** DTaP, Hib, PCV, Rotavirus, Influenza
**Six to 18 months:** DTaP, Hib, PCV, Hepatitis B, IPV, MMR, Varicella, Hepatitis A

**UK Recommended Immunization Schedule:**
**Two months:** DTaP (diptheria, tetanus, and pertussis, or whooping cough), IPV (polio), Hib (haemophilus influenza type B), Hepatitis B, PCV (pneumococcal disease), MenB (meningococcal B), Rotavirus
**Three months:** DTaP, IPV, Hib, HepB, Rotavirus
**Four months:** DTaP, IPV, Hib, HepB, PCV, MenB
**12 to 13 months:** Hib, Meningitis C, PCV, MMR, MenB booster

# Postpartum depression

A woman's hormones remain all over the place after the birth of a child, so it's hardly surprising that some new mothers get what's known as the baby blues. They can cause mood swings, affect her sleeping patterns, and make her cry for no reason. Fortunately, they normally pass after a few weeks.

But dads need to watch out for something much more severe— a psychiatric disorder called postpartum depression (PPD), or postnatal depression. It affects around 10 percent of mothers but, unchecked, it can cause major problems for baby, mother, and you, too. Extreme symptoms include rejection of the baby, irritability, lack of concentration, anxiety, crying, anger, sadness, guilt, loss of interest in friends and hobbies, sleeping problems, exhaustion, loss of appetite, headaches, stomach ache, and sore muscles. Make sure she gets medical attention.

In very rare cases, new mothers can suffer from an extreme psychological disorder known as postpartum, or postnatal, psychosis. Symptoms can be devastating—hallucinations, paranoia, mania, delusions, and suicidal impulses. It's crucial to seek medical attention straightaway, since a woman suffering from this disorder might attempt suicide or harm the baby.

# Dads get baby blues, too

It's true. A study by the National Childbirth Trust in the UK revealed more than one in three dads are concerned about their mental health. Not every dad is instantly filled with love for his new child. But unlike maternal postpartum depression, the paternal version is caused by social factors, such as a fear of fatherhood, financial worries, resentment at the death of his social and sex life, and jealousy of the baby.

Yes, it may sound childish, but a father's jealousy of his newborn is totally understandable. The sudden mutation from husband or boyfriend to father can be an unsettling process. Yesterday you were the light of your partner's life. Today you seem like an irrelevance. In one fell swoop, you've been demoted to the bottom of the family hierarchy.

The truth is—and few fathers will admit to this—that paternal love isn't always instinctive. Sometimes it has to be learned. For many dads, a newborn baby can be a stranger who dominates the mother, disrupts sleep, and cries constantly. Sometimes it's not until the baby starts to interact, recognize his father, smile even, that the father is really drawn to him. Many dads take several months to fall in love with their child.

# Baby transport

Don't scrimp on baby transport. Unless you plan on holing up with your baby in the living room for the next four years, you need a high-quality stroller, baby carrier, and car seat. Baby transport is like your own set of wheels: yes, in theory, you can survive with a cheap, worn out old wreck but life is so much more pleasant with a pricey SUV.

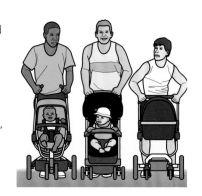

Nowadays, all baby transport is rigorously checked for health and safety issues. Keep an eye out, however, for rough edges, sharp points, and exposed hinges. You can guarantee your baby will put his fingers where he shouldn't.

## Choose the right system

Think about what kind of traveling you're going to be doing with your baby. Will you be spending a lot of time in the car? Do you live in a city center with well-groomed sidewalks, or will you be crossing rough terrain? New York Subway? London Underground? City buses? Are you sporty? Do you plan to jog with your baby buggy? Will you be transporting your baby on your back? Where are you going to store the buggy in your house? All these factors need to be considered before you buy.

**Slings:** Ranging from basic slings to more sophisticated versions, these wrap the baby to the mother. Perfect for hippy dads, too.

**Baby carriers:** With adjustable harnesses, these are designed to attach either to your back or your front. For use around town, the front-attached ones are better, since you can protect your baby from getting bumped into. But if you're out hiking in the country, you'll need a carrier that attaches to your back. Look for storage pockets for changing materials.

**Car seats:** Baby car seats normally come with a protective overhead bar that doubles up as a carrying handle. With infant car seats, your baby can sit upright and you can strap him in racing-car style. Choose a seat that's simple to secure and adjust, or you risk giving yourself a coronary every time you attempt to clip in the safety belt. Try an ISOFIX/LATCH base that anchors directly to the car's body. This allows you to secure and remove the car seat easily. Great when taking a sleeping baby out the car.

**Classic prams:** Don't be old-fashioned. These Victorian designs may be efficient, but you're a modern dad. Also, they become pointless once your baby can sit up.

**Basic Strollers:** Lightweight and mostly cheap, these are great for taking on public transport or on vacation. Some even offer a reclining seat for babies. But they're rarely sturdy enough to withstand the rigors of daily baby life. And

you can't take them off-road. Perhaps keep one as your second buggy at Grandma and Grandpa's.

**All-terrain strollers:** These are great for active parents. Featuring portable bassinets for babies, proper seats for toddlers, pneumatic tires, and storage compartments, they are designed for any baby transport dilemma. Some of them you can even take out jogging.

**Double strollers:** Planning a second baby? Got twins? You need a double stroller. Opt for tandem rather than side-by-side style, they're far more maneuverable.

**Complete travel systems:** Super-versatile, these feature a portable bassinet-cum-car seat that attaches to a stroller base. Again, ideal for moving a sleeping baby directly from car to stroller without waking him up.

**Child seats for bikes:** Your baby will need to be able to sit on his own before using these. They come either front- or rear-mounted. The former are better for really young toddlers, the latter for older kids. He'll need his own helmet.

# Form filling and thinking ahead

Assuming you are not a criminal on the run from the authorities or an anarchist determined not to let "the man" tell him what to do, you will want to carry out the necessary legal procedures required when you have a baby. That means it's time to get your new baby into the system and to plan for his future security. Inevitably, there's a bit of paperwork, and with everything that's going on, it may be tempting to put these tasks to one side, but don't leave it too long.

**Registering your baby** In the USA, depending on which state your baby is born in, the hospital will give you the relevant paperwork, which is then sent on to the state authorities for registration.

In the UK, all babies must be registered within 42 days of their birth (21 days for those born in Scotland). You can do this either in the hospital before the mother leaves, or at the local registry office.

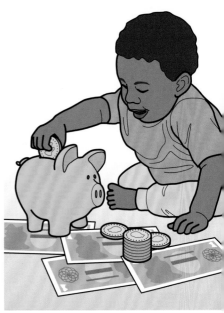

**Making a will** You're no longer the reckless, carefree soul you used to be. A tiny being now relies on you and your partner for everything. That's why you both need to draw up a will.

Your will should state who is to receive your money, real

estate, vehicles, and valuables in the event of your death. You can designate who your child's legal guardian will be, should you and his mother die before he comes of age, and who will manage money and assets on his behalf.

If money is tight, you can check online and draw up a do-it-yourself will, but it's easy to make mistakes—much better to hire a legal expert and get it done properly.

● Make a list of all your bank accounts, real estate, investments, life insurance, and expensive valuables.

● Most parents arrange their wills so that their partner inherits everything if one dies, while their child inherits everything if they both die.

● Designate who your child's guardian will be.

● Designate who will manage your money and assets.

● Choose an executor to manage the paperwork after your death.

● Decide what type of funeral you would like.

**Investing for your baby** This book certainly isn't about investment advice. However, it's worth thinking about your child's financial future as early as possible. Depending on which country you live in, there are various opportunities to invest money for your newborn in savings accounts. You can encourage family and friends to give him money at birthdays and Christmas. By the time he reaches 18, he'll have a nice little nest fund. Your job then will be to persuade him not to blow it all on a sportscar.

**Life insurance** Last year, you could have popped your clogs and life would have trundled on quite happily. Right now, though, a little person is relying on you. Get life insurance so that, should you die, he'll be well looked after.

# The stay-at-home dad

Choose this role and you're in a very small minority, but in the western world at least, it's a minority that is growing every day. In the US, the percentage of at-home dads has risen from 1.6% in 2001 to 3.4% in 2011. A recent study by a UK insurance company stated that the father was the main carer in one out of seven UK families. It's normally for financial reasons that fathers stay at home to look after the baby, but there are other factors, such as the ability to take a career sabbatical or work from home, that make the decision to defy convention more appealing. Think of yourself as unique.

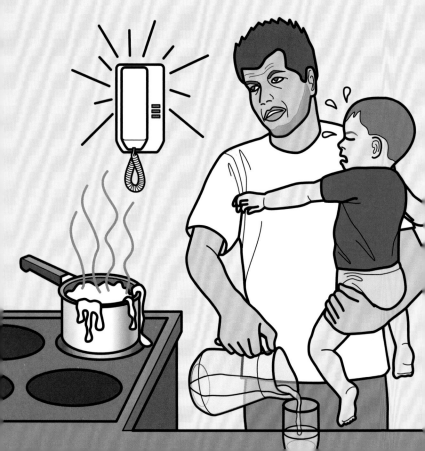

**Learn how to multitask** Ever tried to get dressed and cook breakfast at the same time? For many women, this is a cinch. For men, such multitasking can be impossible. However, all stay-at-home dads need to become multitasking experts. You can practice the skill by using multitasking tools, such as a hands-free phone or a front-mounted baby carrier. Playpens, baby bouncers, and baby seats will keep the little one occupied on his own for at least a few minutes.

**Ask for help** Grandparents, neighbors, friends, babysitters … they can all help you out when things become crazy. When your partner gets home, you don't need to mention that you required the services of a wingman. Baby certainly won't squeal.

**Join a support group** In both the USA and the UK, plenty of support groups are there for stay-at-home dads. If there is a local group you can join, then why not give it a try? Men sometimes shy away from these groups, but they can be very useful for sharing experiences of fatherhood or even just talking about the latest sports results. If you're at home five days a week with only a four-month-old for company, you'll be glad of any conversation you can get.

**Part-time work** Many stay-at-home dads also have part-time jobs. Provided you're not leading a secret second life, it's always better to be honest with your employers and let them know you are juggling caring for your child with work. They may even admire you for your multitasking skills.

**Get outside** The one advantage you have over new mothers is that you are physically stronger. This means you can be more mobile. Simply strap your baby into a front-mounted baby carrier and head off to the park or playground. (See page 80.)

**Ignore the sexism** As a male homemaker, you are bound to be on the receiving end of a certain amount of sexism. Mothers may assume you're not up to the job or that the baby's mother has left you. Fathers may think you've thrown away your career or that you've lost your job. Treat sexism as a challenge. Your mates are likely to give you a bit of grief as well, but remember that they are only teasing and you can be confident that the bond you develop with your child will be considerably stronger than if you were out at work all day.

**Encourage independence** The more you encourage your baby to fend for himself, the easier your job becomes. That doesn't mean you can let him get the bus home on his own, but a bit of solo toy-play will get him used to being on his own occasionally.

**Picnics** Babies demand food every few hours. And if they don't get it, they quickly become very grumpy, which means if you want a day out with your baby, you need to take lots of supplies (see below).

## Packing for a day out

Heading out for the day with a baby is a major military operation that requires a bit of planning. Don't underestimate the time it takes to prepare all the supplies needed for a successful few hours outside the house—there's nothing worse than being 5 miles from home and realizing you've left the diapers in the bedroom or the baby formula in a bottle in the refrigerator. Leave getting him dressed until last, particularly if you are in a hurry; that way, you will avoid having to deal with a last-minute poop in the diaper. Carry everything you need in a backpack so that your hands are kept free to deal with any situations. Alternatively, most baby strollers will have a handy shelf underneath where you can store all the essentials.

**Baby transport (see page 80):** When he's very young, keep things simple by using a baby carrier. You'll be much more maneuverable.

**Diaper-changing gear:** Think how many diapers you'll need for the whole day and then double the quantity. Don't forget wipes, diaper bags, and changing mat.

**Provisions:** You'll need food and milk, beaker and spoon, and bibs.

**Toys:** They're great if they clip onto your baby carrier or stroller.

**A change of clothes:** You'll be on the bus and suddenly there's poo all the way up his back and down his legs.

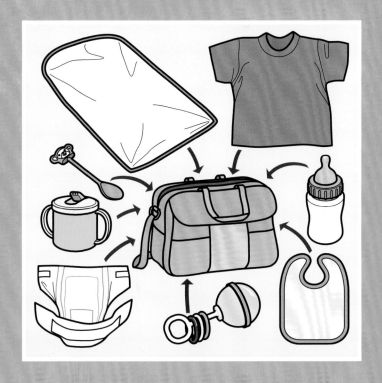

# When does your sex life resume?

Things have no doubt been a bit lean recently. While you may now be champing at the bit, the last thing on your partner's mind will be sex. Few women will want even to consider the idea until six weeks after the birth. Some prefer to wait longer. Besides, it's likely been a bit of a car crash down below, and she will want to be sure everything is healed and back to normal. Lack of sleep, breastfeeding, and jumbled hormones will further bury her sex drive. When she does eventually want to get things going again, you'll have to be extra gentle. And remember that a demanding baby means recreation time in the bedroom will be a lot less spontaneous.

While breastfeeding women are unlikely to be ovulating, it is still possible for them to get pregnant. In your haste to revive your sex life, don't forget about contraception. You think one baby is a handful? Imagine having two under two years old.

# Baby first aid

It's not a bad idea to take a baby first-aid course. You'll learn how to deal with everything from burns and bruises to choking and meninigitis. But with or without this expert knowledge, it's a good idea to keep a baby first-aid kit in the house— somewhere easily accessible for you but well out of reach of inquisitive fingers.

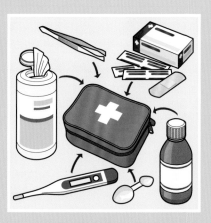

# First-aid kit essentials

● Band-Aids (cartoon characters are popular)

● Antiseptic wipes and cream

● Baby acetaminophen (Tylenol or paracetamol) or ibuprofen

● Thermometer (see page 69)

● Medicine spoon

● Tweezers

● Insect repellent

● Calamine lotion (for insect bites or rashes)

● Cold pack (for bumps and bruises)

● Baby electrolyte solution (for diarrhea dehydration)

# Baby CPR

CPR, or cardiopulmonary resuscitation, can save the life of a baby who has stopped breathing.

Make sure someone has called the paramedics and then place the baby on a firm, flat surface. Remove any obstructions from his mouth. Now you need to give him what's known as rescue breaths. Place your mouth over both his nose and mouth and blow five steady breaths. Repeat this sequence five times.

If this doesn't cause his chest to rise and he doesn't start breathing, you need to do chest compressions. Using two fingers, push firmly straight down 30 times on his breastbone. Then give him two more rescue breaths. Repeat this cycle until he starts breathing again or the paramedics arrive.

# Common ailments

Here are a few common mishaps that can happen to babies.

**Bumps and bruises:** Keep an ice pack in the freezer. Like Band-Aids, cartoon-character ice packs are popular. Frozen peas will suffice. If it's a head bump, watch out for signs of concussion (drowsiness, vomiting), in which case, head for hospital.

**Nose bleeds:** Lean your baby slightly forward as he's sitting in your lap. Pinch the bottom of his nose gently shut and wait until the bleeding stops.

**Choking:** Babies can't resist putting things in their mouths, and that's pretty much anything. Your job, as Dad, is to be vigilant and make sure it's nothing small enough to choke on.

If there's something blocking his airway and making him cough, it's best to let him continue coughing, since this may dislodge the object. If it doesn't, lie him face down along your arm (his head lower than his chest) and, with the heel of your other hand, strike him firmly five times between the shoulder blades to dislodge the object. If this doesn't work, turn him onto his back and, using two fingers, push firmly inward and upward five times on his breastbone. Meanwhile, someone should be calling an ambulance.

**Burns:** For anything but a minor first-degree burn, you should get medical treatment. A first-degree burn is when just the outer layer of skin is damaged. Treat this by holding the burned area under running cold water for ten minutes. Then dry the skin and cover it with a sterile bandage. If the burn starts to blister, seek medical attention.

**Bee and wasp stings:** Scrape the little black sting off your baby's skin with a fingernail. Squeezing it releases more poison. Apply an ice pack to reduce the swelling. If he's six months or older, use children's antihistamine, which you can buy from the drugstore.

# Traveling abroad with babies

If you and your partner are longing for a vacation, what's stopping you? While a trip to the Amazonian rainforest may not be the best idea, there's no reason why you shouldn't travel abroad with your little one. Besides, he won't have any school commitments and most airlines will transport him for free on your lap. Make the most of it.

Even newborns need their own passports, so get the admin done well before you're due to fly. Be warned—there are a lot of bureaucratic hoops to jump through (mainly to prevent child abduction). For American babies, visit www.travel.state.gov; for British babies, visit www.gov.uk.

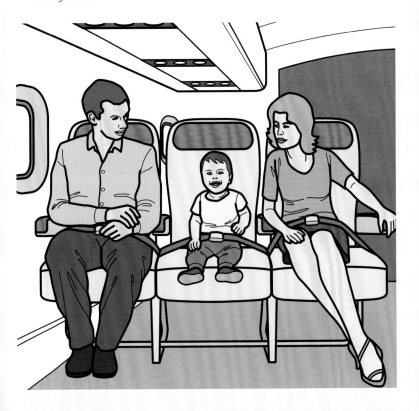

# Baby and daddy play

This is a great way to bond with your little one. He will get plenty of cuddles from both of you but one area where you, as father, can really excel is with rough-and-tumble play. Put some music on, scatter loads of cushions around the living room, and get active with your baby. Bounce him up in the air, roll him around, tickle him. As he develops physically, encourage him to turn over onto his tummy, then to crawl, then to stand. Don't beat yourself up if he shows no interest in walking.

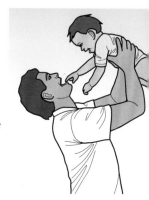

Keep the entertainment simple, though. A six-month-old has no interest in traipsing around a dusty old museum (unless it's particularly baby-friendly, see page 95); nor does he wish to learn letters and numbers. Be realistic—ten minutes of peekaboo and a leisurely stroll around the backyard should suffice.

**Toys:** Within a few weeks of your baby's birth, you will find yourself knee-deep in plastic toys. Where do they come from? Do the toys breed with each other? Is it a Chinese conspiracy to take over the world?

Much of this plastic is utter rubbish. A two-month-old baby will derive just as much pleasure from a saucepan and a wooden spoon as he will from the latest Disney figurines. Much better to spend your money on toys that will improve his physical development.

**Baby gyms:** These are perfect for a newborn who can't yet crawl. He lies on his back on the padded mat while the overhanging toys keep him amused.

**Baby bouncers:** Another great amusement for a pre-crawler, baby bouncers are a classic diversion. He bounces in the chair while playing with the rack of toys suspended in front of him.

**Doorway jumpers:** You put him in the seat and attach the elastic ropes to the top of the doorway, letting him bounce. Be warned, though. Some medical experts believe they can adversely affect a baby's physical development.

**Playpens:** At last you can turn your back on him for a few minutes. Fill the playpen with toys and he will amuse himself for hours. For some older babies, playpens may seem like jail, though. Offer him parole if he needs it.

**Activity walkers:** For a crawling baby, you can get a walker that allows him to sit in a seat and push himself around with his feet. For one who is just beginning to walk, try a contraption a bit like Grandpa's walking frame, which will support him as he wobbles along. All types come with panels of various toys attached.

**TV:** For some parents, sitting a baby in front of the TV is tantamount to teaching him how to smoke. In any case, newborns can't tell the difference between the evening news and "Sesame Street." But sometimes the bright lights and colors on the screen will keep him amused long enough for you to go for a pee or have a shower.

## Mental stimulation

Calculus and Dostoyevsky are a little bit advanced right now, but there's no reason why you shouldn't start stimulating your baby mentally from the very start. Talk to him, repeat easy words and the names of objects, read books to him—touchy-feely ones are great, as are those with noisy buttons—and sing songs to him.

# Great baby days out

With all the constant baby care, your partner will really appreciate some time off from the little one. Why not organize a baby and daddy excursion? As long as he has progressed to bottle-feeding, you'll cope perfectly well on your own. But you'll need to plan your day with military precision. (See page 86 on packing for a day out.)

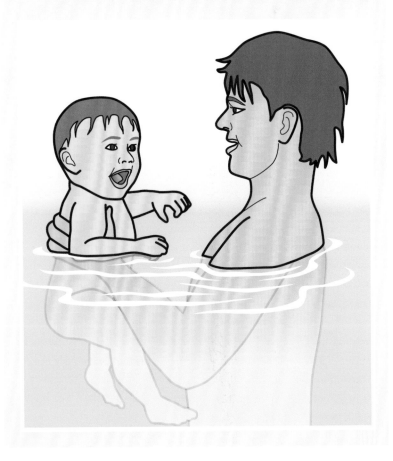

## Park

It's great to expose your baby to nature. He'll love lunchtime picnics, with a big rug for him to crawl on. Just keep an eye out for dog poo. If it's there, your baby is sure to locate it and stick his fingers in it—like a moth to the flame.

## Playgrounds

While most playgrounds are designed for toddlers and older, as long as he can support his head, there are some rides you can help him on.

## Libraries

Of course he can't read yet. But many libraries have a baby section with touchy-feely books, giving you time to hunt out the latest Grisham novel. Some libraries even run free baby groups.

## Museums

Many museums have interactive areas for the little ones. Even if he doesn't quite grasp the intricacies of an internal combustion engine, he will enjoy pushing the buttons. And it's free to get him in.

## Swimming

Babies love to be splashed about in the water. Just don't lose your grip as you bounce him around, and don't forget the swim diaper. Nothing clears a pool quicker than an errant baby poo. Once he can support his head, you can safely put him in an inflatable baby float.

## Zoos and petting farms

You won't believe how much fun babies can get from stroking furry mammals. At children's zoos and petting farms, there are thousands of these critters to keep them amused. Just make sure you disinfect your hands and your baby's regularly. Most zoos and farms now provide disinfecters.

## Blowing bubbles

You've had a late night. Perhaps you've got a raging hangover. But it's your turn to look after baby. Get out in the yard and blow some bubbles. This activity provides maximum amusement for minimum effort.

# Teething

Any time your baby starts crying, grumbling, or is particularly grouchy, friends and passers-by will helpfully try to tell you it's because he's teething. That's certainly not always the case (see Baby meltdowns, page 76), but teeth emerging from his little gums can understandably be quite a painful experience.

While there are no hard-and-fast rules as to when baby teeth (also referred to as milk teeth and deciduous teeth by dentists) will start to emerge, his first tooth will probably appear when he's between four and seven months old. The initial tooth is likely to be one of the lower middle ones, followed by the upper middle ones. These are known as the central incisors. Next come the two teeth on either side of the middle teeth, the lateral incisors, with the rest gradually emerging as he grows. On average, by the time a baby is three years old, all 20 teeth will have arrived.

The teeth of some babies won't appear until they are 12 months or older, so don't panic if it takes longer than you expect for the first signs of growth to appear—you won't need to start researching false teeth just yet.

The problem with teething is that it makes babies really grumpy. They drool, sometimes so much that the front of their T-shirt gets wet through; all that saliva causes a rash; their gums swell; they find it difficult to sleep or feed; and they bite down on anything in sight—pacifiers, toys, your fingers. Some parents believe teething causes diarrhea and fever, although there's no scientific evidence to back this up.

To relieve his pain, give him something to chew on. Teething rings are good, especially the ones you put in the freezer. So are teething biscuits, frozen vegetables, and cold drinking water. If the pain is extreme—and he'll certainly let you know—you can smooth on teething gel, and give him baby acetaminophen (Tylenol or paracetamol) or ibuprofen. (Check the age restrictions.)

# Baby grooming

**Nails:** Wait until your baby is asleep. That way he'll keep still while you cut his toenails and fingernails.

**Ears and nose:** Use absorbent cotton wool to clean away ear wax and snot. There will be tons of the latter. You may need to wet the cotton so as to soften the snot.

**Teeth:** Even if he has just a couple of teeth, it's important to start cleaning them from a young age. Make sure you do it gently and with a toothbrush and toothpaste specially designed for babies. Baby toothpaste tends to be low in fluoride or fluoride-free. Babies often swallow toothpaste by accident and large quantities of fluoride can poison them. Try to teach them to spit it out.

**Hair:** During the first year you, shouldn't have too many problems with your baby's hair. It grows much quicker on some babies than others, though. Just let it grow. It's not like he's going to a job interview any time soon.

# Moving on to solids (weaning)

Time to redecorate the kitchen? Don't worry, once you switch to solids, your baby will happily do it for you. Before you know it, there will be mashed banana across the kitchen cabinet, up the walls, even on the ceiling. A word of warning—never, ever attempt to feed your baby while you are wearing a suit … unless it's a bio-hazard suit. If you've ever witnessed feeding time at the monkey house, you'll have an idea of what's in store.

For most babies, the time to introduce solid food into their diet is when they are between four and six months old. Before that, your baby's digestive system and kidneys won't be able to handle the onslaught. Both the World Health Organization and the American Academy of Pediatrics recommend that babies are exclusively breastfed until six months old. But some will show signs of needing solids from the age of four months.

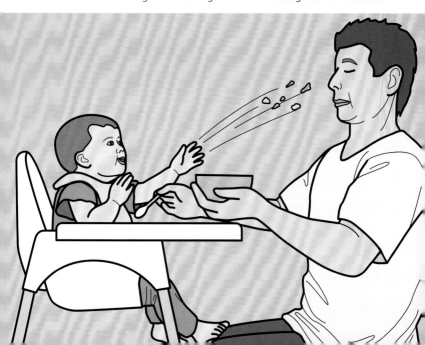

# When is your baby ready for solids?

- He has doubled his birth weight.

- He's at least four months old.

- He can sit up by himself and keep his head in a steady position.

- He's getting lots of milk at regular intervals throughout the day but he still seems hungry.

- He wakes up during the night or early in the morning, clearly hungry.

- He no longer has what's known as the extrusion reflex. Young babies use their tongues to push objects out of their mouths. You won't get any food in there until this reflex fades.

- He shows interest in what you're eating and reaches for your food.

# Start off slowly

After he's had his milk feed—even solid-eaters still need milk until they're one year old—try him out with a few teaspoons of puréed food. Making fresh puréed food at home is surprisingly simple (see page 100), so avoid that processed stuff they sell in supermarkets. Try fruit or vegetables, such as peaches, pears, bananas, sweet potatoes, squash, carrots, zucchini, kiwi fruit, melons, avocados, and peas, and baby rice. You'll need something to mash the food. Food processors are good but electric hand blenders will suffice. Even a fork works, given enough elbow grease.

Once he's happy with the veggie stuff, you might progress to cereals, bread, pasta, fish, meat, pasteurized cheese, raw fruit, berries, and sweet corn. However, there are some foods you should avoid (see page 101). Use a soft plastic spoon so he doesn't hurt his gums. You'll also need plastic bowls, sippy cups, and bibs. To keep them sterile, wash them in the dishwasher on the hot setting. And, remember, you'll need to persevere—babies take a while to get used to the idea of solid food in their mouths. At first he will eat once a day. By eight months that should increase to three times a day. You'll know he's full once he starts clamping up his mouth or turning his head away. Or when he starts redecorating the kitchen.

# On the menu

The best baby food is the stuff you make yourself, but you won't have time to spend hours slaving over a hot stove, only to see your culinary masterpiece splattered across the floor. So here are a few dad-friendly creative shortcuts.

For economies of scale, make batches of cooked, puréed fruit and veg, and freeze it in small portions. You can defrost and combine these portions when preparing meals at a later date.

## Quick, healthy food for six-month- to nine-month-olds

### Mashed banana and avocado
Skin them and mash them together. (Great for when you're out and about.)

### Chicken, sweet potato, and carrot purée
Chop all three ingredients into small cubes. Simmer in salt-free vegetable stock. Once soft, mash into a purée.

### Jacket potato with cheese
Cook a jacket potato in the microwave (it takes around six minutes, depending on the size). Scoop out the potato and mash it with cheese.

### Poached white fish
Poach a white fish in milk until it starts to flake. Flake the fish, removing any bones, even tiny ones. Make a white sauce by adding corn starch (cornflour) to the milk.

# Quick, healthy food for nine-month- to 12-month-olds

### Pasta with tomato sauce
Boil pasta stars until they're soft and mix them with a pot of baby tomato pasta sauce.

### Cornflake fish fingers
Cut a skinned salmon fillet into small chunks (watch out for bones). Dip the chunks into a beaten egg and then coat them with crushed cornflakes. Cook in the oven for 15 minutes.

### Creamy chicken risotto
Fry chopped chicken pieces in a spalsh of olive oil for five minutes. Add risotto rice and frozen peas and gradually mix in salt-free vegetable stock, stirring regularly until the rice is really soft. Stir in a spoonful of cream cheese.

### Eggy bread
Dip finger-sized pieces of bread (crusts removed) into a bowl of beaten eggs. Fry on both sides until they're golden.

## Bad baby foods

While you may pride yourself on having guts of steel, your newborn baby's insides are a little more delicate, to say the least. Once you get him onto solids, you need to be aware that, aside from the obvious, such as fiery Mexican dishes, certain foods need to be approached with caution.

**Salt:** Food with a high salt content isn't good for babies' kidneys.
**Sugar:** Avoid sugary snacks and drinks.
**Honey:** Sometimes honey contains a bacteria that can cause infant botulism. He should be at least one year old before he eats honey.

**Saturated fat:** Avoid foods high in saturated fat, such as potato chips, French fries, and cakes.

**Peanuts:** There's a theory that feeding peanuts to babies can lead to peanut allergies later in life. It's not proven but better safe than sorry.

**Raw shellfish:** This carries a risk of serious food poisoning.

**Shark, swordfish, or marlin:** Possible high levels of mercury in these fish can damage a baby's nervous system.

**Undercooked eggs:** Raw or lightly cooked eggs may cause food poisoning, but well-cooked eggs, that is if both white and yolk are solid, are fine from six months up.

# Choosing a highchair

When Bub first moves on to solids, you can sit him in a bouncy chair or a car seat to feed him. But once he's happily sitting upright, you'll need to invest in a highchair. As ever, the options are endless. Here are a few pointers.

**Plastic highchair:** They're ugly but they're really practical, since they wipe clean easily and feature a tray that keeps spillages all in one place (in theory). If you have a small kitchen, choose one that folds away easily.

**Wooden high chair:** They might match your kitchen cabinets but they tend not to come with a tray, so you have to position your baby at the dining table.

**Booster seat:** These strap to a normal dining chair—not great if you value the upholstery on your dining chair.

**Hook-on chair:** These clamp onto the table top, suspending your baby on the edge of the table. Great if you have a small kitchen, and easily transported if you're visiting friends.

# Childproofing the house

Once your baby starts to crawl, you'll suddenly notice what a deathtrap your house is. It's positively bristling with lethal objects with which he can potentially lacerate/impale/maim/burn himself. Watch him roam around the house and you'll wonder how we ever managed to evolve into the planet's dominant species. Don't be paranoid but take some sensible precautions.

**Smoke detectors:** In a fire, they'll save your life, too. Make sure you test them regularly to see if the battery is still working.

**Baby-proof latches:** Install these onto all the kitchen cupboard doors. They're fiddly and they annoy the hell out of adults but they'll stop him from trapping his fingers in the doors or shattering your favorite china on the kitchen floor … and then crawling across it.

**Cleaning products:** Keep these locked away in a secure cabinet, well out of reach of your baby. Babies can't distinguish water from bleach.

**Medicine:** Same goes for medicine. To a baby, Valium and Viagra look no different from Skittles and M&Ms.

**Electrical socket guards:** They stop little fingers going where they shouldn't.

**Window latches:** Like 1970s rock stars, who seemed to be irresistibly drawn to windows, especially when bearing TV sets, babies don't understand the dangers of defenestration.

**Check for wires:** If he can't reach up to pull your $1,000 PC off the desk, he can still yank on the wires. Tuck them all away.

**Stair gates:** Stairs are fun. To a crawling baby, stairs present a challenge. But babies rarely make it more than halfway up—or down—before gravity takes over. That means you need safety gates at both the base and the summit of your stairs. Some models screw into the walls (much safer at the top of stairs), while others use springs to stay in place. The latter can be moved around the house or taken on visits to the grandparents' place.

# Professional childcare

Parents can't possibly dedicate themselves 100 percent to their baby's early years. Sooner or later, one of you is going to have to go back to work. What if you both have to? You'll need to consider childcare. Here are your options.

**Daycare center (or nursery, as the British call it):** Expensive but highly professional. Your baby will learn to socialize with other babies from a young age. The major downside is that he will pick up every bug imaginable— the spit and snot in a daycare center is like something out of a horror movie—which, in turn, means you will pick up every bug imaginable. Most centers will charge you if you pick up your baby late.

**Home daycare providers (or childminders, as the British call them):** Although your baby will be in someone else's private home, he will still have other babies to play with. Good for parents with uncertain working hours.

**Private nanny:** This tends to be the most expensive option of all. Your baby's safe in your home but has no other little ones to play with. The required paperwork and taxes aren't fun, either.

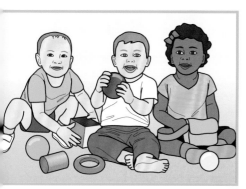

**Live-in au pair:** Less expensive than a private nanny but, of course, you need a spare room. And a willingness to share your house with a 19-year-old.

**Granny:** If you can't trust Granny, who can you trust? And it's free.

# Bad parents

We can't all be perfect fathers. Sometimes it's just too tempting to drown out the sound of crying by turning up the stereo. Here we examine the antics of some of the world's well-known bad dads (and a few moms). Let it be a lesson to all of us.

## Michael Jackson (balcony-dangler)

May the Prince of Pop rest in peace. Just as soon as he's explained why he needed to dangle his youngest son off a fourth-floor balcony in Berlin.

## Britney Spears (baby behind the wheel)

She once famously drove her SUV with her four-month-old son, Sean Preston, on her lap. Her excuse was that she was fleeing the paparazzi.

## Joan Crawford (daughter-shearer)

The Hollywood actress's daughter said her mother once caught her putting on make-up. Her punishment was to have her hair cut off.

## Eddie Murphy (daughter-ignorer)

This *Beverly Hills Cop* sired a daughter with Spice Girl Mel B but refused to acknowledge either mother or child. He now pays child support.

## Danniella Westbrook (cocaine at childbirth)

The British soap star admitted on TV that she took cocaine during the birth of her son.

## Arnold Schwarzenegger (adulterer)

The Governator admitted that he sired a lovechild with the housekeeper while his wife was pregnant.

## Woody Allen (stepdaughter-lover)

He married his own stepdaughter. Enough said.

## Music for babies

However dedicated a parent you are, there are only so many times you can endure "The Wheels on the Bus," To keep junior amused—and also retain your sanity—you need to compile some music that both you and he will love. Catchy choruses and repetitive verses work well, as do lyrics about animals, mommies, and daddies. You'll need upbeat songs for the daytime; lullabies for bedtime.

## Top ten cool (and cheesy) baby and daddy tunes:

1. Sweet Child O' Mine by Guns 'N' Roses
2. Baby, I Love You by The Ramones
3. Daddy Cool by Boney M.
4. De Do Do Do, De Da Da Da by The Police
5. Yellow Submarine by The Beatles
6. Walking on Sunshine by Katrina and the Waves
7. You Are the Sunshine of My Life by Stevie Wonder
8. Three Little Birds by Bob Marley & The Wailers
9. Dream a Little Dream of Me by The Mamas and The Papas
10. Love Me Tender by Elvis Presley

# Troubleshooting for babies

Babies don't come with a manufacturer's guarantee. You can't take them back when they go faulty. And they will go faulty at some point. But there are a few tricks of the trade you can use to keep them happy.

### Problem: Baby won't stop crying

**Solution:** Find the reason and you'll find the solution. He's hungry, he's tired, he's ill, he's hot, he's cold, he's bored, he wants to be cuddled, he's got wind, he's teething, you've accidentally stepped on his finger.

### Problem: Baby's teething

**Solution:** Use teething rings, teething biscuits, frozen vegetables, or cold water. In extreme cases, use teething gel and give him baby acetaminophen (paracetamol) or ibuprofen.

### Problem: Baby won't eat

**Solution:** Fly a spoonful of food around the room like an airplane, eventually landing in his mouth.

### Problem: Baby's coughing all the time

**Solution:** If he's got colic, massage his tummy or use baby medicines, such as Infacol. If he's got croup, it will pass. If he's got whooping cough, take him to the doctor, who will probably give him antibiotics.

### Problem: Baby's got diaper rash

**Solution:** Apply a barrier cream (zinc oxide- or petroleum-jelly-based) or a diaper-rash cream. Plenty of brands are available.

### Problem: Baby's got diarrhea

**Solution:** Keep him hydrated. If he's not also throwing up, give him milk. If he is, get a pediatric electrolyte solution from the drugstore.

### Problem: Baby's got eczema

**Solution:** Use soap-free body wash and emollient skin cream.

# Baby facts

For the next 12 months at least, conversation with your partner and friends will rarely stray from the subject of babies. While you may be dying to talk about sport, music, politics—anything other than the bowel movements of an infant—you're going to have to accept that your newborn will be the default topic. So why not arm yourself with all the coolest facts and figures about pregnancy and babies? You'll be the life and soul of any dinner party.

## Number of babies
Four million babies are born in the USA ever year; 790,000 in the UK.

## Place of birth
In the USA, 99 percent of births take place in hospital; 0.6 percent at home; 0.3 percent in birth centers. In the UK, an average of 2.5% of births take place in the home each year.

## Date of birth
Most American babies are born on a Tuesday, fewest on a Saturday. (That may be because C-sections rarely take place at weekends.) Most babies are born in late summer; obviously, couples like to cuddle up during the cold winter months.

## C-section
A third of American babies come out the sunroof; a quarter of British babies arrive that way.

## Gender
In both the US and the UK, 105 baby boys are born to every 100 baby girls. That's bad news for over-protective dads.

# Weight

The average weight of an American newborn is 8lb (3.6kg); for a British baby it's 7lb 5oz (3.3kg). The largest baby ever born was a staggering 23lb (10.4kg)—that must have hurt.

# Multiples

A Russian woman in the 17th century is said to have given birth to 69 children, including 16 pairs of twins, seven sets of triplets, and a set of quadruplets.

# Youngest mother

In 1939, a five-year-old Peruvian girl gave birth to a baby boy by C-section. Her dad was later arrested for incest.

# Smallest baby

The smallest recorded baby ever born weighed just 8.6oz (244g) and was 10 inches (25cm ) long.

# Pregnant man

The prize goes to American Thomas Beatie who, in 2008, became the world's first "legally pregnant" man to give birth—whatever that means. The transgender male has since had two more kids.

# Stay-at-home dads

According to recent United States census data, the number of men who are the primary carer for their children has risen to around 626,000. Numbers in the UK have also grown, to around 227,000.

# PART 4

# SOME FRIENDLY ADVICE

Fast forward to a year after your child is born and you could be forgiven for thinking there's a global conspiracy against new fathers—it's definitely not always like you see in the movies. No one warns you that there's a good chance that your carefully planned water birth accompanied by the soothing sounds of whale song won't actually happen. People keep quite about the fact that gas and air offers little in the way of pain relief—it doesn't do much for the mother, either—or that you may need to stay in the hospital for a few nights once the baby is born. You're of course aware of the sleepless nights but you had no idea a baby could cry non-stop for 78 hours. Post-baby blues—what are they all about? And why did nobody mention that your inability to produce breast milk can sometimes make you feel completely redundant when faced with a screaming infant? These are the aspects of parenthood that, for some reason, no one tells you about. To compensate for this conspiracy of silence, we have brought together some first-hand accounts from real fathers who have lived through childbirth and child rearing, and have survived to tell the tale. Be warned, they pull no punches. However, we hope that by sharing these stories they will demonstrate that although things often do not go according to plan, it's highly likely that everything will work out absolutely fine in the end. And nothing can beat the feeling of seeing your baby smile for the first time.

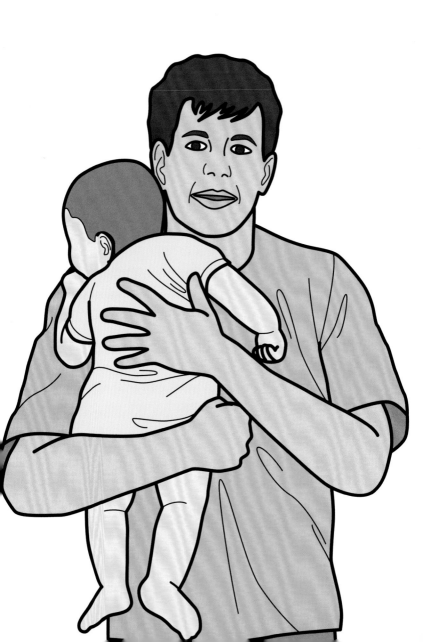

# Warnings from the pregnancy

## It's not just your partner tha can be affected by hormones

**During his wife's pregnancy, in 2013, Damien started noticing some very strange hormonal changes… but in his own body rather than his pregnant partner's.**

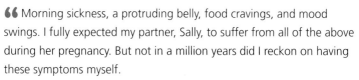

❝ Morning sickness, a protruding belly, food cravings, and mood swings. I fully expected my partner, Sally, to suffer from all of the above during her pregnancy. But not in a million years did I reckon on having these symptoms myself.

Sure enough, about three months into Sally's pregnancy, just as she was really starting to show all the usual physical and psychological signs, my body decided to join in sympathy with hers. I started to feel major shifts in my moods. On more than a few mornings, I felt nauseous—and it was nothing to do with a hangover. But things got really bizarre when I noticed my belly sticking out much further than usual, protruding just like Sally's, and then I began to crave fast foods such as burgers and fried chicken. Normally I'd steer well clear of fattening stuff like that.

Naturally, I went to see my doctor who told me I was probably suffering from a phenomenon known as Couvade Syndrome. It's not a recognized medical condition but apparently it's more common than you'd think. Some experts believe it's psychosomatic, caused by men worrying about their partner's pregnancy, or trying somehow to empathize with their partner's condition; or even some weird kind of pregnancy envy.

Whatever the reasons, it wasn't much fun. We already had quite enough to worry about with Sally's pregnancy. We certainly didn't need both of us waddling around the house, feeling sick and miserable, and eating like a person possessed. Fortunately my body stopped short of causing my breasts to grow. Apparently it's rare but it's not unknown for men suffering from Couvade Syndrome to experience swollen breasts and even fluid from the nipples. Yowzers!

The day after Sally gave birth to a very healthy eight-pound baby girl, my symptoms disappeared in an instant. It was quite bizarre. It just proves how the whole thing must have been psychosomatic. And, thank God, I never showed signs of lactating.**"**

## Beware unexpected changes in your partner's personality

**In 2015, Paul and his partner Zoe were expecting their first child. What Paul wasn't expecting was Zoe's sudden insistence on turning their home into the perfect baby palace.**

**"** Apparently they call it the 'nesting instinct.' But, until my partner, Zoe, was six months into her first pregnancy, I'd never before heard of this phenomenon. I wish someone had warned me about it.

Zoe is one of the most relaxed and calm people I know. Nothing normally fazes her. But, six months into her pregnancy, all she could focus on was making our house spotlessly clean, and turning our spare room into the picture-perfect nursery. She changed from being really laid back to being utterly obsessive. It was the total change in character that really threw me.

Our baby was due in mid-February. Around November time, a full three months before the birth, our conversations continually revolved around redecorating our spare room and making it perfect for the baby. I don't actually recall talking about much else. I was playing it cool, reassuring her there were still three months to go until the baby was due. For Zoe, nothing else mattered.

I told her I had a friend who would redecorate the room for us. So, every morning she would ask me if I'd booked him in to do the job. And she started planning the décor of the room—with all the zeal of a professional interior designer. We didn't know the sex of the baby so we had to choose gender-neutral color schemes and wallpaper. I kid you not, I must have looked at a couple of thousand wallpaper patterns before we eventually managed to agree that pictures of little birds were suitably non-gender specific.

Zoe got pretty fed up with my lack of a sense of urgency. She couldn't understand why I didn't share her need to feather the nest. And I got frustrated with the fact she wasn't her normal chilled self. Soon she gave up on my promises to get my decorator friend in and hired her own handyman herself. As well as the baby's room, the rest of the house had to be prepared, too: everything was polished, tidied, dusted, cleaned, sometimes twice a day. You know something unusual is going on when your partner gets up at 6am on a Sunday to wipe down the skirting boards.

Then Zoe started researching strollers and baby buggies. In my usual laid-back way, I'd planned simply to buy one a couple of weeks before the birth. But Zoe was far more organized than that. Months before the birth she was online and in the shopping mall, checking out the different models on offer. She also decided she ought to learn how to drive. Having avoided it thus far in her life, she took lessons and quickly passed her test. It was another part of the nesting procedure, I suppose. **99**

# Rules for the birth

## Have a birth plan, but don't be surprised if you have to abandon it

**Archie and his wife Maria had their second child Jake in 2008. During the birth, just about everything that could go wrong did go wrong.**

❝ My wife had been in labor for 15 hours so she was pretty exhausted by the time the baby started emerging. Unfortunately, the maternity unit failed to spot just how big the baby was. They should have suggested a Cesarean, but instead they decided to force him out the normal way. They were using a ventouse (a rounded cup applied to the baby's head) and forceps; there was lots of blood; it was horrendous.

There was a particularly wonderful moment when the doctor had his ventouse attached to Jake's head, and one foot up against my wife's bed in order to get proper purchase. He was pulling like mad. Suddenly the vacuum suction in the ventouse was released and it swiftly came off Jake's head. The doctor flew back across the room, poleaxed himself against the opposite wall, smashed his head, and was then promptly showered in blood flying out of my wife's vagina. You could not make this stuff up.

In the end, because Jake was already halfway down the birth canal, they couldn't opt for the plan B of a Cesarean. Instead they were forced to administer an epidural and slice Maria open to get him out. She was losing so much blood. We eventually got Jake out but the maternity team were so busy dealing with the new-born that they failed to notice Maria had stopped breathing and gone blue. I screamed at them to turn their attention to her. Then we had a situation where half the team were working on her while the other half looked after the baby. There were eight medical people in there, in all, too many to fit comfortably in the room: three doctors, plus various nurses and midwives.

I didn't think I was going to lose Jake but toward the end I did think Maria was in serious trouble. She was in that hospital recovering with Jake for close to a week afterwards. He was born weighing 10 and a half pounds—that's a seriously big baby. We gave him the middle name of Kipling because it means 'salmon,' and I once caught a salmon of a similar weight. **"**

## You might not make it to the hospital

**In 2011, Jake and his wife Emma were expecting their second baby. Traffic wasn't good that day.**

**"** It's safe to say that my wife Emma is a complete control freak. But she also has an irrational fear of hospitals and medical procedures. With that in mind, she and I planned the birth of our second child, Olivia, with military precision. Every single little detail had been considered: overnight bags were packed, the fuel tank of the car was full, our phones were charged, Granny was on standby to look after our older child, an aunt was available as a back-up, and we knew the route to our hospital like the back of our hands. What we hadn't accounted for were the vagaries of Mother Nature.

The problem was Emma didn't actually realize she was going into labor until it was too late. She wasn't feeling uncomfortable in the slightest. We had been out for the day and when we got home it caught us entirely by surprise. Before I knew it, she was kneeling down in the bathroom, immoveable. Try as I might, I couldn't get her out of the bathroom. There was no way I was going to get her downstairs on my own. Manhandling her into the car and off to hospital was out of the question.

To add to our problems, half an hour after we'd telephoned Granny, she was still nowhere to be seen. It turned out she'd had a minor car accident on the way over to our house.

Five minutes later, the doorbell rang and I rushed down to answer it, thinking it was the back-up aunt. What do I find? A homeless person knocking on our door asking to shelter from the rainstorm. I was pretty sure he had no medical qualifications so I swiftly turned him away.

Because of the rainstorm, the aunt was also delayed—stuck in traffic. So I did what any normal person would do: I panicked and called an ambulance.

Fortunately the ambulance arrived fairly quickly. Unfortunately neither of the two paramedics in it had much experience delivering babies. One had helped bring a baby into the world a couple of years previously. The other barely knew what a new-born baby looked like. But, give them their dues, they somehow managed to carry Emma from the bathroom to the bedroom, and planted her on the bed. Minutes later Olivia was born. Sadly the mattress was ruined but, aside from that, things proceeded fairly well. The paramedics were brilliant.

Later, the midwife arrived from the hospital to see us. Mother and baby were signed off and, within a couple of hours, we were all three downstairs, toasting the baby's health with a glass of champagne.**99**

# A baby can turn up when you least expect it

**Perhaps rather unwisely, Andy headed off to play a round of golf when, in 2005, his wife Pippa was close to giving birth to their second child.**

**66** Confident that my heavily pregnant wife would be fine, I left for a day's golf at a lovely club 30 miles from home. I joked with my friends that I was chancing things a bit. But, to be honest, the golf was not to be missed.

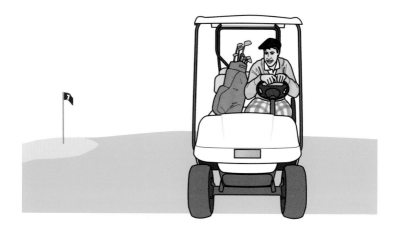

On the seventh hole, about as far from the clubhouse as you can get, my phone suddenly rang. It was my mother-in-law saying she was taking her daughter to the hospital as the waters had broken. Fortunately we managed to commandeer a golf buggy from an elderly gentleman on a neighboring hole, and I was driven quickly back to the clubhouse. I threw my clubs in the back of the car, tore off out of the car park, and then the blinking light on the fuel gauge of my Honda Accord caught my attention. A quick mental calculation told me that it was 35 miles to the hospital, so I should just about make it. I pressed on.

What about the speed restrictions, though? My reasoning was that if I was stopped by the police for speeding, they would surely understand my actions. At one point I was at nearly double the speed limit, and the fuel-gauge needle was well below zero.

On the final run to the hospital there were half a dozen traffic lights that all went against me. As I slowed to stop at one of them, the car made a grinding sound as if the exhaust had just collapsed. I was so close to the hospital that I figured it was best to press on and check later.

On arrival at the maternity unit, just 42 minutes after receiving the call from my mother-in-law, I couldn't resist a quick look under the car to see what had caused all the noise: the under tray of the engine had collapsed and was dragging on the road. Still, I'd arrived there in one piece, without running out of fuel or being jailed for speeding. I was able to join my lovely wife for the final throes of her labor—a reasonably quick affair which culminated in the birth of our son, Ted.

At that point one of the midwives noticed I was still wearing my studded Footjoy golf shoes. She told me it was appropriate footwear, given the mess of afterbirth that I was standing in.

Now 10 years old, my son is happy and healthy and able to confidently strike a golf ball. He also has a fascination with fast cars. My wife is happy as I have since given up golf.**"**

## If this is not your first child, don't count on the birth being like the previous one

**Dino and his wife Helen were expecting their third child in December 2008. By now fully experienced in the birthing process, they weren't anticipating any hiccups. The only slight problem was that the baby was scheduled to arrive on December 25th.**

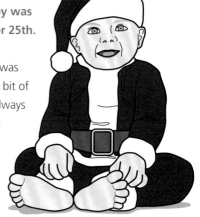

**"** When the doctors told us Sofia was due on Christmas Day, we all had a bit of a laugh. In my experience, babies always arrive later than predicted, so in my mind, we were looking at a birth date around New Year's Eve.

But Santa Claus had other plans. Sure enough, early on

Christmas morning, about 7.30am, just as I'd given our other kids their breakfast, Helen started going into labor.

Her previous births had taken a ridiculously long 18 hours or so, which meant I wasn't panicking at all. In fact, as her contractions started, I was taking it very easy, casually putting my shoes on, thinking about a leisurely drive to the hospital.

Suddenly, bang! Her waters broke right there in our front hallway. Being Christmas, my parents-in-law were staying with us. While I was helping Helen ease down to the ground, my father-in-law was straight on the phone requesting an ambulance. I wouldn't be surprised if Helen's screaming woke up the entire street on that Christmas morning.

The paramedics arrived 12 minutes later, and two minutes after that, the baby started to appear. Only one of the paramedics had time to get in through our front door before it all kicked off. He told me to fetch some old towels (by then it was a bit late for all that) and then placed his hands strategically to hold the baby as it came out. It was his first job of Christmas Day, and it was his first baby delivery ever. My poor father-in-law, on the other hand, saw more of his daughter than any dad ought to.

For various reasons to do with my wife's blood group, we had to then wait for the midwife to arrive before we could cut the umbilical cord. Then, a bit later, Helen attempted to stand up. It was all a bit much for her and she passed out momentarily so the paramedics decided to take her to hospital to keep an eye on her. I followed in our car with Sofia in the baby seat.

When we eventually got home from the hospital on Christmas Day evening, I was so exhausted that I told Helen I'd just whip up a quick plate of pasta for both of us. 'No you won't,' she told me quick as a flash. 'We've bought all the stuff for the Christmas dinner and you're now going to prepare the lot.'

So I had to cook the whole meal for everyone. Turkey and everything. Having not eaten all day, Helen was by then ravenous. **"**

# A lot of births have complications, but the experts can work miracles

**Lee had a traumatic experience with the birth of his third child, in 2013, but it all turned out okay in the end.**

❝ After two easy hospital births, we decided to have a home birth for our third child. Unfortunately, at the last minute the midwife noticed the baby was breech. My wife, Arla, was quickly rushed to hospital in an ambulance.

The minute we arrived, the baby started coming out, legs and bottom first. This is when things started to go very wrong. Basically the baby got stuck with her neck and head still inside the womb but the rest of her body dangling out.

Within seconds there were suddenly 20 medical people in the room. I had this out-of-body experience; everything around me went into slow motion. I thought the worst.

The midwife turned to Arla and said 'You have got to push right now'. So she did, and our daughter, Mary-Jane, finally came out. But she was gray and limp. I honestly thought she was dead. All the medical people were going crazy.

I crouched down to peer between all these people and see what the hell was going on. I saw a doctor put his fingers down my daughter's throat, pull her head back and start pumping oxygen inside her. Then they started resuscitating her, but nothing was happening. She was motionless for a total of nine minutes.

I thought, 'That's it, she's gone.' I was in severe shock.

Then suddenly I saw her little diaphragm move up and down slightly. I nearly fell onto the floor at that point. But I assumed our baby would be brain damaged from lack of oxygen. I later discovered that new-born babies are actually able to survive this lack of oxygen for some time.

Mary-Jane was immediately transferred to intensive care where a nurse said to me: 'It's what we do now that determines whether she will come through unscathed. This is the bit where we save her life.' The tears were rolling down my cheeks as I realized we weren't yet out of the woods.

After five days in intensive care Mary-Jane finally started putting on weight and transformed from this tiny gray being into a normal-looking baby. It was miraculous.

We now have a beautiful, healthy child. Because my wife hadn't seen what I'd seen, she adapted very quickly. I, on the other hand, was quite traumatized by the whole experience.

What struck me most was that I had assumed everything would be plain sailing with our third baby because we'd had two uneventful births before Mary-Jane. This experience taught me that's not always the case. **99**

# Advice on baby care

## Never forget your baby

Gordon, and his wife Marina couldn't wait to go out for the first time after the birth of their baby. It had been ages since they'd properly socialized with anyone.

❝ Our baby George was just ten weeks old. We'd successfully negotiated the really tough stuff: the gruesome early diaper changes, the totally sleepless nights, the utter confusion of a new parent. Finally, we were starting to see a chink of light at the end of the tunnel. Miracle upon miracle: George was now actually sleeping for four hours stretches. Not long now and we might get our social lives back.

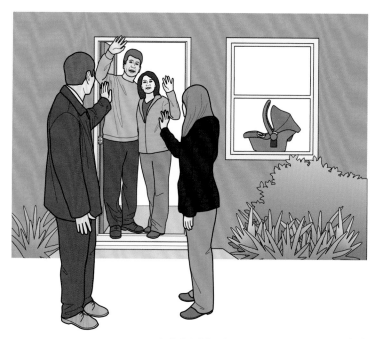

Our first proper invitation out was to a friend's dinner party on the other side of town. George was still too young to leave with a babysitter so we asked our friends if we could bring a travel cot and put him to sleep in their spare room while we ate with them. No problem. We could even get there early and give him a wash in their bath. It seemed like the perfect set-up.

We duly remembered to bring all the paraphernalia we'd need before we could relax and enjoy the dinner party. We took several changes of clothes, the baby basin for the bath, the baby soap, the travel cot, and, of course, the baby monitor so that we wouldn't have to leave the dinner table every three minutes to check on the little one.

Finally, after about an hour and half of baby duties, we got George to sleep and went downstairs to the party. The whole evening went swimmingly. Inevitably much of the conversation centered around George and his various activities, as it always does when new parents come to a dinner party. The wine was flowing liberally. We both had a drink or two—nothing silly but enough to celebrate the fact that our social lives were not, as we had once feared, over. In fact, we were the last couple to leave the party.

We were about halfway home (as designated driver, I'd held back on the wine), when suddenly my phone rang. It was the host. 'Do you think you might have forgotten something?' he said, suppressing a laugh.

I slammed on the brakes and turned to my slightly inebriated wife. 'We've only gone and left George asleep in their spare room,' I told her as she looked at me in abject horror.

In the years since, our dinner party hosts have never allowed us to forget that incident of child neglect. Neither have any of the other guests from the same evening. In fact, pretty much everyone I've ever known has been told this story. **99**

# Traveling with kids is not easy

**Matt had to travel abroad quite a bit with his baby Grace during her first year. It wasn't always easy.**

❝ Flying with babies is never pleasant, but unsympathetic fellow passengers make it much worse. First off, there's the humiliation of having to dismantle the stroller at the boarding gate, and feeling the hateful glare of the other passengers when you are given priority boarding. Then you see them silently praying they won't be sitting anywhere near you.

I remember one flight we took with Grace from London to Pisa, in Italy. This grumpy old man was sitting in the seat row in front of us—you know the type. All throughout the flight, as Grace was gurgling and crying, he kept turning round, tutting at us, and berating us for not keeping our baby silent. Just as we were preparing for landing, he said to me: 'I don't really think Pisa is the place to take a baby!'

Any parent who decides to travel by air with a baby needs to have thick skin. Let's face it: you'll never be popular. The best you can hope for is that other passengers treat you and your baby as if you are suffering from Ebola. They won't want to sit anywhere near you, they'll regard you with suspicion, and they'll hold their breath any time you approach.

I've paid my dues with baby travel over the years, spending hours trying to entertain Grace on flights only to be rewarded with exploding vomit all over my lap. As a flying new dad, you quickly learn to bring spare clothes for both you and your baby. Here are some other top tips:

● Always bring an iPad—it's the best baby distraction tool on the planet.

● Never take your state-of-the-art stroller abroad with you. Instead, buy a really cheap one from the thrift store or charity shop. They're lighter, smaller, and they won't clog up the waiter's path in overseas restaurants.

● Pack really light. Once you've filled your suitcase with all the baby paraphernalia, you quickly realize you've only got room for one spare T-shirt and pair of underpants. Count yourself lucky. ❞

# Useful websites

Here's a list of websites that are great resources for expectant dads and new fathers:

**Baby Center**
An extensive parenting website with sections aimed at dads as well as mothers.
www.babycenter.com

**Centers for Disease Control and Prevention**
Provides information from the US Department of Health on immunizations for babies.
www.cdc.gov/vaccines

**Dad.Info**
Run by the Family Matters Institute, this site delivers over 2 million pages of information to dads each year.
www.dad.info

**Dads Adventure**
Lots of advice and articles on this website specifically aimed at dads.
www.dadsadventure.com

**DIY Father**
Provides practical parenting information, from pregnancy through to teenage years.
www.diyfather.com

**Fathers.com**
Run by the US National Center for Fathering and aimed at helping dads become good fathers.
www.fathers.com

**FQ**
A magazine aimed at dads that also has an excellent website.
www.fqmagazine.co.uk

**Great Dad**
A parenting resource written from the dad's point of view.
www.greatdad.com

**Minti**
An active parenting community site with thousands of articles and advice given by other parents.
www.minti.com

**New Dad's Survival Guide**
A handy site for dads-to-be presented by Bounty, the UK's largest parenting club.
www.newdadssurvivalguide.com

**NHS Pregnancy and Baby**
An excellent site, run by the UK's National Health Service, covering every aspect of having a baby.
www.nhs.co.uk/conditions/pregnancy-and-baby

**Stay At Home Dads**
Sound advice and information for men who take care of their kids.
www.stayathomedads.co.uk

# Index